EXTENDING

SAS® Survival Analysis
Techniques for Medical Research

Alan Cantor

Comments or Questions?

The author assumes complete responsibility for the technical accuracy of the content of this book. If you have any questions or comments about the material in this book, please write to the author at this address:

> SAS Institute Inc.
> Books by Users
> Attn: *author's name*
> SAS Campus Drive
> Cary, NC 27513

If you prefer, you can send email to sasbbu@unx with "comments for *author's name*" as the subject line, or you can fax the Books by Users program at (919) 677-4444.

Table of Contents

Preface

This is a wonderful time to be involved in medical research. One reason is the explosion of knowledge that our colleagues in the basic biological sciences are creating. We are experiencing a constant stream of new discoveries that have the potential to expand our understanding of the causes, prevention, amelioration, and treatment of human disease. But, because human beings are such complex organisms, results from the basic sciences can rarely, if ever, be sufficient to allow us to be certain of the application of these discoveries to humans. Thus, the accomplishments of the basic scientists inevitably lead to exciting and potentially beneficial research projects for those of us who are involved in such activities.

Another reason for the above statement is that never before have we had a greater ability to collect and organize data from our research and to subject those data to the type of detailed and powerful analyses needed to address our studies' questions. A good argument can be made that the increase in our ability to compute and manipulate data, which we have seen within the lifetimes of many of us, surpasses by several orders of magnitude the increases that technology has provided in other areas of our lives.

To say that this computational power enables us to do our work much faster is to vastly understate its importance. In fact, it makes it possible for us to consider and use analytic techniques that, only decades ago, would have been considered much too labor intensive to be worthwhile even if they had been introduced in statistical journals.

Consider just one example in this book: in Chapter 4, "Proportional Hazards Regression," you will find a discussion of the Cox Regression method and an example of the use of that method to study the effects of seven characteristics on the disease-free survival of patients with melanoma. Using the Cox Regression method, as this example does, requires the inversion of matrices of dimension seven. In fact, it requires several such matrix inversions. Now, I know how to do such matrix inversions in theory. I learned about that several years ago when I was a student. For class exercises, we did it for some three dimensional matrices, and we might have inverted a four dimensional matrix inversion or two. Even with calculators (this was in the 1960's), that was all anyone could really expect. If an investigator in 1972 had read Cox's classic paper introducing his method and asked me to use it on some of his data, I undoubtably would have explained to him that it was a theoretically interesting approach, but not practical. By contrast, I now do such things all the time. The example referred to at the beginning of this paragraph was accomplished with two or three minutes of my time—the time it took to type in a few lines of SAS code—and a few seconds of computer time. It was done not on some mighty university or government-based mainframe, but on a desktop computer in my home. Indeed, such computers have become consumer items commonly sold in electronics shops and discount stores.

It is important to recognize, however, that when discussing computational power, the computer itself is only part of the story. The other, perhaps more important part, is software. To return to the example of the previous paragraph, during the 1970's many research institutions had computers that were suffiiciently powerful to perform the calculations required by the Cox Regression method. However, there were no generally available programs to do it. Thus, if a researcher had wanted to use this method to analyze his data, he would have had to obtain access to his organization's computer and write a program to do so. Such a program would probably have been written in an early version of FORTRAN or BASIC, two popular algebraic languages. There were probably some research organizations at which someone had written such a program for his or her colleagues to use. If you were at one of them, or could otherwise obtain a copy of the program, you could use the method. Otherwise, you were out of luck.

The point is that an article in a journal describing a new and powerful statistical technique is often only the first step in that technique's being added to the armamentarium of researchers. Unless and until software to implement the technique becomes widely disseminated, it is unlikely to gain wide use or acceptance. It is for this reason that software companies such as SAS Institute have come to have such an important place in all of those research areas, including medicine, that require statistics. The fact is that not only the statistical methods used in such areas, but also the manner in which they are implemented and results presented, are often determined by which of these methods are implemented by software companies and by the details of those implementations.

This is also the reason that I have chosen to include, in this book, several macros which implement methods (described in the biostatistical literature) that I have found useful in my own work. In some cases these capabilities, as far as I know, are not yet widely available in any other fashion. In other cases they are available from other sources, but I feel that my macros might be more useful. Because power and sample size calculations are very important when planning clinical trials, I include several macros for this purpose.

I would be remiss if I did not issue a warning concerning the potential for misuse of the vast computational power provided to us by modern computers and software. This power is, indeed, a double-edged sword. In the "old days," when computation was difficult, we would think very hard about what analyses to do. If different approaches were possible, we would decide in advance what made the most sense in our particular situation. Today, such prior thought is often considered unnecessary and therefore, is not practiced. It is so easy to produce vast amounts of analyses that it is tempting to look at our data in every way we can think of, rather than in the way that makes the most sense. If there is more than one valid method of testing an hypothesis, we might do all of them rather than deciding in advance which is most appropriate. Such practices can not only cause considerable confusion, but also lead to invalid conclusions.

Still another unfortunate consequence of the power provided by modern computational resources is that it is no longer necessary for a user of statistical techniques to have any understanding of the results obtained as a result of their use. In the 1970's, a statistician who wrote a FORTRAN program for doing Cox Regression could hardly avoid understanding what the results meant. However, anyone can mimic an example found in the SAS software documentation and submit, as a SAS job, the following:

```
proc phreg;
model time*cens(0)=x y z;
run;
```

Being able to do that in no way guarantees that the user will understand what the output means and the assumptions under which the results are valid. You are urged to consider these issues when using the methods described in this book and in SAS documentation.

The first chapter of this book, "What Is Survival Analysis?", introduces you to survival-type data. The first thing you need to understand is what makes such data special and why a class of methods dealing specifically with survival-type data is needed. Why not, you might ask, simply use more standard methods? For example, why not compare survival times in two groups by a pooled *t* test? The basic problem with that, and what creates the requirement for special methods, is the possible existence of subjects who have not died at the time the analyses are being performed. This chapter introduces the terminology to be used thoughout the remainder of the book and describes some alternative types of functions that can be used to describe survival. All of this will be needed in the remaining chapters.

In the interest of uniformity of language in this book, methods are described using words like "mortality" and "death." It is important that you realize that these methods are equally applicable for the time until the occurrence of any well defined endpoint. In medical research, this might be recurrence of disease, the development of toxicity to a treatment, or remission of symptoms. In fact, survival methods have been used in non-medical research areas as well. The time until a someone who is released from prison commits another crime, the time until a light bulb fails, or the time it takes a child to master the multiplication tables, are three such examples. As a consequence of my background, the examples and terminogy used in this book are from the medical sciences; however, I hope that readers with major interests in other areas will find this book helpful as well.

Chapter 2, "Nonparametric Survival Function Estimation," discusses the most commonly used nonparametric method of estimating survival rates at various times, the Kaplan-Meier method. The LIFETEST procedure, described in that chapter, can be used to perform this method. A pair of macros are also given, KMTABLE and KMPLOT, which offer certain capabilities that are not found in PROC LIFETEST. As with other problems in estimation, it is often useful, when planning a study, to be able to choose a sample size that will result in a standard error small enough to assure reasonable precision of the estimate. A macro that does that, KMPLAN, is also given.

Chapter 3, "Nonparametric Comparison of Survival Distributions," continues the discussion of nonparametric methods. In this chapter, the focus is on the comparison of groups. The LIFETEST procedure does this using the two most commonly used techniques for this purpose, the log rank test and the Wilcoxon (also known as the Gehan) test. These tests are actually just two realizations of a rather broad class of tests, known as linear rank tests. The LINRANK macro is offered here to provide greater flexibility in choosing the test statistic you want to be used. Another macro, POWER, can be used to calculate the power of each of these tests under various assumptions. This macro can thus guide the choice of test statistic.

Chapter 4, "Proportional Hazards Regression," discusses the Cox Proportional Hazards Regression method and the SAS procedure, PHREG, that performs it. This technique has become extremely popular in medical literature, especially since it has become available in commercial software products such as SAS software. It is especially useful for describing the joint effect of various covariates on survival. Because "treatment group" can be one of those covariates, it can be used to compare two (or more) treatments as an alternative to PROC LIFETEST. Unfortunately, it is often used without understanding its underlying assumptions or the meaning of its results. For these reasons, I have a lot to say about these matters in this chapter.

Sample size and power considerations are important here as well. However, because of the complexity of the model when several covariates are considered, this is feasible only when the number of covariates does not exceed two. A macro for that purpose is given.

Chapter 5 discusses parametric methods. These methods can provide the greatest amount of information about the survival function and how it is influenced by various covariates of interest. SAS provides a procedure, LIFEREG, that performs this analysis for certain types of parametric models. A more general macro, PARAMEST, is also given and described in this chapter. For example, an analysis using this macro might indicate that certain risk factors have positive or negative impacts on the probability of cure while others impact on the survival time of those test subjects who are not cured. Particular attention is paid, in this chapter, to estimation of cure rates. This can be thought of as the limit of the function giving the probability of surviving until time t as t increases without bound. In many situations, the proportion of subjects who are cured is of much greater interest than the proportion of those who survive two or three years.

Although these methods are most informative, that information is always somewhat clouded by the realization that its validity is conditioned on the chosen parametric model being at least approximately correct. The issue of whether to use parametric or nonparametric methods is, of course, not limited to survival methods. It is a persistent problem. Everyone who does statistical analyses frequently has had to decide whether to use a pooled t test (parametric) or a Wilcoxon Rank Sum test (nonparametric), or whether to compute the Peason correlation coefficient (parametric) or the Spearman correlation coefficient (nonparametric). The difference is that, in these situations, there is generally only one parametric model to choose—that described by the normal distribution—and the parametric method and the nonparametric method usually produce quite similar results. In survival analyses, however, this is often not the case. We can choose among several parametric models, and the results can be quite model dependent. I offer no easy solution to this problem, but do suggest some graphical ways to check your data for fit to some common parametric models. A macro that does this is given.

Because it is difficult to remember the details of how to invoke these macros, I suggest that you use the templates provided for each. These templates provide the names of the arguments that need to be provided. They also include internal documentation to remind you of what each of these arguments represents. Of course, you don't have to use these templates, but I find them useful and think that you will also. You don't have to type the macros and templates. On the inside of the back cover of this book, you will find instructions on how to download them.

In writing this book, I've tried to keep in mind the needs of several types of readers. For those who wish to use SAS software for survival analyses, but who have little or no previous training in statistics, I hope this book will enable them to produce some useful results. For such readers, I have included some material, usually not included in software-oriented books, on the bases for some of the methods discussed. To avoid interrupting the flow of the discussion of the methods, this material is appended to the ends of the chapters to which they apply. For readers who have backgrounds in statistics, but not in the methods of survival analysis, I've tried to provide a reasonable introduction to the subject. For those who are already knowledgeable in the methods of survival analysis but who have not used SAS software to do them, I hope this book can accelerate the process of becoming proficient in doing survival analysis using SAS software. Finally, for those of you who are already skilled at using SAS to perform survival analyses, I hope you find that the macros are useful and that you are motivated to improve upon them.

This is where authors usually acknowledge and thank all of those who have helped, in one way or another, to produce their book. I don't know where to begin or where to end. So many people have, directly or indirectly, made their contributions. Most didn't even know it. I've been very fortunate to have teachers who shared so much of their knowledge with me, students who inspired me to find more clear ways to explain complex ideas, and colleagues who were generous in giving me the benefit of their experience. Special thanks go to all of the medical researchers that I have worked with over the years for patiently helping me to bridge the gap between the textbook and the real world.

I'm also appreciative of the assistance provided by the folks in the User Publishing Department at SAS Institute. In particular, the book benefitted greatly from perceptive reviews by SAS Institute personnel. Colleagues at the H. Lee Moffitt Cancer Center and Research Institute also provided helpful reviews. Notwithstanding this assistance, any errors are attributable to me alone.

I don't list any names of the individuals referred to here only because I fear that I might produce a lengthy list and still unfairly omit someone. You know who you are, and you have my thanks.

One exception: My heartfelt appreciation to my wonderful wife, Bootsie, for her support, forbearance, and love. Without her, this book would not exist. And that's only the beginning.

Chapter 1   What Is Survival Analysis?

1. The Nature of Survival Data

Survival data are special and, thus, they require special methods for their analyses. Before going into what makes these data special and how they are analyzed, let's establish some terminology and explain what is meant by survival data.

Although you might naturally think of survival data as dealing with the time until death, actually the methods that are discussed in this book can be used for data that deal with the time until the occurrence of any well-defined event. In addition to death, that event can be, for example,

1. Relapse of a patient in whom disease had been in remission.

2. Death from a specific cause.

3. Development of a disease in someone at high risk.

4. Recovery of platelet count after bone marrow transplantation.

5. Relief from headache, rash, nausea, etc.

Note that for examples 1, 2, and 3, longer times until the event occurs are better. For examples 4 and 5, shorter times are better. Nevertheless, the methods that are described in this book can be applied to any of these examples. For the purpose of this book, words like *survival* and *death* are used to describe these methods, but you should be aware of the broader areas of applicability.

This might be a good place for a few words about example 2 on the above list, cause-specific death. When you analyze the survival of patients with, for example, some form of cancer, you might want to focus on death caused by cancer, particularly in an older population in which we expect deaths from other causes as well. You would then count as "events" only those deaths caused by cancer. A death from any other cause would be treated the same as if the patient had suddenly moved out of state and could no longer be followed. Of course, this methodology requires that you establish rules and a mechanism for distinquishing between cause-specific and noncause-specific deaths. In the New York Health Insurance Plan study that was designed to assess the efficacy of mammography (Venet et al. 1988), women were randomized either to a group that received annual mammography or to a group that did not. Since the study's planners realized there would be considerable mortality not related to breast cancer, they took as their endpoint death caused by breast cancer. A committee was created to determine whether or not the death of a woman was due to breast cancer. This committee, which was blinded with respect to the woman's group assignment, followed a detailed algorithm that was described in the study protocol.

What makes analyses of these types of data distinctive is that often there are many subjects in whom the event did not occur during the time that the patient was followed. This can happen for several reasons. Here are some examples:

1. The event of interest is death, but at the time of analysis the patient is still alive.

2. A patient is lost to followup without having experienced the event of interest (death).

3. A competing event occurs that precludes the event of interest. For example, in a study designed to compare two treatments for prostate cancer, the event of interest might be death caused by the cancer. However, a patient might die of an unrelated cause instead, such as an automobile accident.

4. A patient is dropped from the study, without having experienced the event of interest, because of a major protocol violation or for reasons specified by the protocol.

In all of these situations, you don't know the time until the event occurs. Without knowledge of the methods that are described in this book, a researcher might simply exclude such cases. But clearly this throws out a great deal of useful information. In all of these cases, we know that the time to the event was at least some number. For example, a subject who was known to be alive three years into a study and then moved to another state and could no longer be followed is known to have a survival time of at least three years. This subject's time is said to be *right censored*. A subject's observed time, t, is right censored if, after time t, he or she is known to still be alive. Thus you know that this subject's survival time is at least t. A survival time might also be *left censored*. This happens if all that is known about the time to death is that it is less than or equal to some value. A death is *interval censored* if it is known only that it occurred during some time interval. Although much current research focuses on ways to deal with left- and interval-censored data, most survival analytic methods deal only with right-censored data. Of the three SAS procedures that deal explicitly with survival data, two deal only with right censoring. This is the type of censoring most commonly seen in medical research. The third, the LIFEREG procedure, which is discussed in Chapter 5, "Parametric Methods," deals with left and interval censoring as well. Except for that chapter and a section in Chapter 3, this book does not consider left- or interval-censored times, and the term *censored* will always mean *right censored*.

Survival data, therefore, are described by a pair of variables, say (t, d). They can be interpreted as follows:

t represents the time that the subject was observed on study.

d is an indicator variable that specifies whether the event in question either ocurred or did not occur at the end of time t. The value of d might be 0 to indicate that the event did not occur or 1 to indicate that it did. Then $d=0$ means that the corresponding t is a censored time. Of course, you can substitute your choice of values.

The SAS survival analysis procedures, as well as the macros that are presented in this book, do allow the user to specify any set of values to indicate that a time is censored. This is convenient when you have data in which a variable indicating a subject's final status can have several values that indicate censoring. Subscripts will be used to distinguish the subjects. Thus, if there are n subjects in a study, their survival data might be represented by the n pairs $(t_1, d_1), (t_2, d_2), \ldots (t_n, d_n)$.

Sometimes in textbooks or in journal articles, survival data are reported by using only the time variable. Censoring is indicated by adding a plus sign to the time. For example, reporting survival data as 2.6, 3.7+, 4.5, 7.2, 9.8+ would mean that the second and fifth observations are censored and the others are not. In a data set, you can store information about both the survival time and the censoring value using only one variable. Censoring is indicated by making the time negative. Using this convention, the above data would be 2.6, -3.7, 4.5, 7.2, - 9.8. A SAS DATA step can easily be written to convert such a data set to the desired forms, which contains separate variables for t and d. This is illustrated by the example code and output below:

```
proc print data=original;
title 'Original Data Set';
data; set original;
d=1;
if time<0 then do;
        d=0;
        time=-time;
        end;
proc print;
title 'Modified Data Set';
run;
```

```
                    Original Data Set

                 OBS      TIME

                  1        2.6
                  2       -3.7
                  3        4.5
                  4        7.2
                  5       -9.8


                    Modified Data Set

              OBS      TIME     D

               1       2.6      1
               2       3.7      0
               3       4.5      1
               4       7.2      1
               5       9.8      0
```

There is another way of thinking about the variables t and d. Each patient on study is really subject to two random variables: the time until death (or the event of interest) and the time until censoring. Once one of these events happens, you can observe that time but not the other. The variable t can be thought of as the minimum of the time until death and the time until censoring. The variable d indicates whether that minimum is the time until death ($d=1$) or the time until censoring ($d=0$). An important assumption in any analysis that follows is that the time until death and the time until censoring are independent. This would generally be true, for example, if censoring occurred simply because the follow-up period ended. On the other hand, suppose you are analyzing the data from a study in which patients with some sort of cardiac disease are randomized to drug treatment or surgery. In some cases it might later be decided that a patient randomized to drug treatment now needs to get surgery. You might be tempted to take the patient off study with a censored survival time that is equal to the time until surgery. However, if the decision for surgery was based on the patient's deteriorating condition, to do so would create bias in favor of the drug treatment. That is because such a patient's death would not be counted as a death once he had been censored. A better approach might be to anticipate this possibility when planning the study. You might plan the study as a comparison of two treatment strategies: immediate surgery versus initial drug treatment with surgery under certain conditions that are established in advance.

2. Calendar Time and Study Time

Another concept we need to discuss is how time is defined in survival studies. In most survival studies, patients do not all begin their participation at the same time. Instead they are accrued over a period of time. Often they are also followed for a period of time after accrual has ended. Consider a study that starts accrual on February 1, 1996 and accrues for twenty-four months until January 31, 1998 with an additional twelve months of follow-up until January 31, 1999. In other words, no more patients are entered on study after January 31, 1998, and those accrued are followed until January 31, 1999. Now consider the following patients:

Patient #1: Enters on February 15, 1996 and dies on November 8, 1996.

Patient #2: Enters on July 2, 1996 and is censored (lost to follow-up) on April 23, 1997.

Patient #3: Enters on June 5, 1997 and is still alive and censored at the end of the followup period.

Patient #4: Enters on July 13, 1997 and dies on December 12, 1998.

Their experience is shown graphically in Figure 1.1. In survival analyses, all patients are thought of as starting at time 0. Thus, their survival experience can be represented as in Figure 1.2. When reference is made to the number surviving or the number at risk at some time, the time referred to is the time from each patient's study entry–not the time since the study started. For example, among the above four patients, two of them (#3 and #4) are still at risk at 12 months. None are still at risk at 24 months. Both of these statements are made based on Figure 1.2. If, at some later date, you speak of those who are at risk at $t = 6$ months, that has nothing to do with the situation on July 31, 1996, 6 months after the start of the study. Rather you mean those who, as of the last date that the data were updated, had been on study for at least 6 months without dying or being censored.

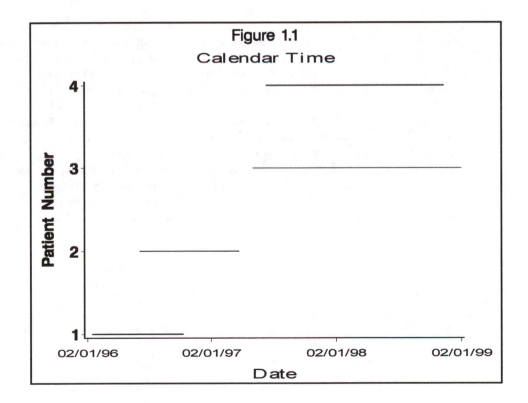

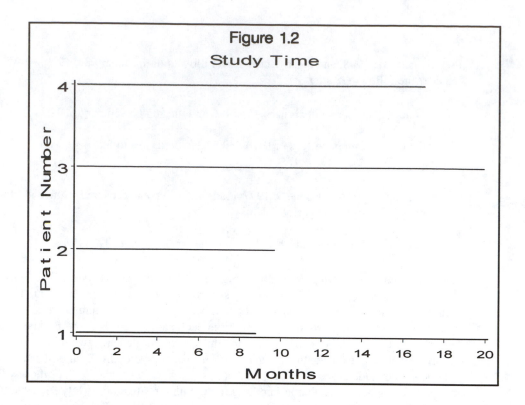

3. An Example

Sometimes in studies that involve follow-up of patients, there is interest in more than one time variable. For example, an oncology study might examine the time until death, which will be called *survival time*, and the time until death or relapse, which will be called *disease-free survival time*. The database must then contain information on both endpoints. Because SAS handles dates internally as numeric constants (the number of days before or after January 1, 1960), it is often convenient for the data sets to contain the dates of interest and to include in a SAS DATA step the statements to calculate the time values that are needed. As an example, consider a sample of patients who are treated for malignant melanoma. Presumably they are rendered disease free surgically. Suppose that, in addition, they are treated with either treatment A or B, both of which are thought to inhibit relapse and improve survival. We might want to consider both survival and disease-free survival of these patients and how they are affected by treatment, tumor thickness, stage of disease, and tumor site. The database might look like this:

PTID	DATESURG	DATEREL	DATEDTH	DATELAST	TRTMENT	SITE	STAGE	THICK
13725	10/5/93	11/6/94	1/5/95	1/5/95	A	1	III	1.23
25422	3/7/93	.	2/6/94	2/6/94	B	3	II	1.13
34721	9/6/94	.	.	3/18/95	B	2	III	2.15
etc.								

Note the inclusion of a unique patient identifying number, PTID. While this number will play no role in the analyses of this data set, it is a good idea to associate such a number with each patient on a trial. This will facilitate merging with other data sets if you decide to add other variables of interest later. Names are usually not good for this purpose because of the risk of spelling variations and errors. Also, note that treatment (TRTMENT), site (SITE), and stage (STAGE) are represented by codes or brief symbolic names. For obvious reasons, we should avoid having long words or phrases for things like disease site or tumor histology. TRTMENT is a dichotomous variable. Although numbers are used for the possible sites, SITE is categorical. The numbers used do not imply any ordering. STAGE is ordinal; stages I, II, III, and IV represent successively more extensive disease. Finally, tumor thickness in millimeters (THICK) is a continuous variable. Later chapters discuss SAS procedures that deal with all of these types of variables. In this case, missing values for date variables are used to indicate that the event did not occur. In order to analyze survival time and disease-free survival time, the following variables are needed:

DFSEVENT has the value 1 if the patient died or relapsed, 0 otherwise.

DFSTIME is the time, in months, from surgery to death or relapse, if either occurred. Otherwise, it is the time that the patient was observed after surgery.

SUREVENT has the value 1 if the patient died, 0 otherwise.

SURVTIME is the time, in months, from surgery to death, if the patient died. Otherwise, it is the time that the patient was observed after surgery.

To add the variables that are needed to analyze survival and disease-free survival to the data set, the code might look like this:

```
data melanoma; set melanoma;

   /*  Defining dfs time and event variables  */
dfsevent = 1 - (daterel = .)*(datedth = .);
   /*  Divide by 30.4 to convert from days to months */
if dfsevent = 0 then dfstime = (datelast - datesurg)/30.4;
else dfstime = (min(daterel, datedth) - datesurg)/30.4;
```

```
/* Defining survival time and event variables */
surevent = (datedth ne .);
if surevent = 0 then survtime = (datelast - datesurg)/30.4;
else survtime = (datedth-datesurg)/30.4;
```

The divisions by 30.4 are simply to convert time from days to months, a more convenient time unit. Note that 30.4 is approximately 365/12. Also, when terms such as (daterel=.) or (datedth=.) are used in an arithmetic expression, they have the value 0 if false and 1 if true. The above statements create the variables DFSTIME and DFSEVENT to be used in analyses of disease-free survival, and the variables SURVTIME and SUREVENT to be used in analyses of survival. The first three observations of the resultant data set would look like this:

```
PTID  DATESURG  DATEREL   DATEDTH   DATELAST  TRTMENT  SITE STAGE

13725 10/05/93  11/06/94  01/05/95  01/05/95     A       1   III
25422 03/07/93  .         02/06/94  02/06/94     B       3   II
34721 09/06/94  .         .         03/18/95     B       2   III

     PTID   THICK   DFSEVENT   DFSTIME   SUREVENT   SURVTIME

    13725   1.23       1       13.0592      1       15.0329
    25422   1.13       1       11.0526      1       11.0526
    34721   2.15       0        6.3487      0        6.3487
```

Now that these variables have been defined, there are several questions you might want to address. For example, using the methods described in Chapter 2, "Nonparametric Survival Function Estimation," you might want to estimate the survival and disease-free survival probabilities over time for the overall cohort and for subgroups defined by treatment, stage, site, etc. Standard errors and confidence intervals for those estimates can also be calculated. You might also want to perform statistical tests to assess the evidence for the superiority of one treatment over the other. This is discussed in Chapter 3, "Nonparametric Comparison of Survival Distributions." Now, it might happen that the patients who were treated with treatment A had a worse prognosis (as seen by their stages, perhaps) than did those treated with treatment B. If the treatment assignment was not randomized, this might happen if the treating physicians preferred treatment A for more advanced tumors. Even if the treatment assignment were randomized, it could happen by chance that one of the treatment groups had a higher proportion of patients with more advanced disease. Using methods that are discussed in Chapter 3 and in Chapter 4, "Proportional Hazards Regression," you will learn how to compare the two treatments after adjusting for the stage of the disease. In addition, you will be able, if you make certain assumptions, to create a model that produces estimated survival and disease-free survival probabilities for patients with specified values of the above variables. Techniques for doing this are presented in Chapters 4 and 5. For example, you will learn how to estimate the probability that a patient will survive for at least three years if that patient is treated with treatment A for a stage II tumor of thickness 1.5 mm at site 1.

4. Functions that Describe Survival

4.1 The Distribution Function and the Survival Function

The survival time of a subject being followed on a clinical study will be thought of as a random variable, T. As with random variables in other areas of statistics, this random variable can be characterized by its cumulative distribution function, often simply called *distribution function*, denoted $F(t)$ and defined by

$$F(t) = Pr[T < t], \ t \geq 0 \tag{1}$$

That is, for any nonnegative value of t, $F(t)$ is the probability that survival time will be less than t. Of course, you could just as well describe the random variable, T, in terms of the probability that survival time will be at least t. This function is called the *survival function* and will be denoted $S(t)$. We then have

$$S(t) = 1 - F(t) = Pr[T \geq t], \ t \geq 0. \tag{2}$$

By convention, $S(t)$ is usually used in survival analysis, although $F(t)$ is more commonly used in other areas of statistics.

4.2 The Density Function

Another function that is useful in describing a random variable is the *density function*. To understand how this function is defined, think of the change in the value of a cumulative distribution function (as defined in the previous section) as t increases by a small amount, say from t to $t + \Delta t$. Symbolically, this change can be written as $F(t + \Delta t) - F(t)$. The average change over the interval is simply this value divided by the interval length, that is

$$\frac{F(t + \Delta t) - F(t)}{\Delta t} \tag{3}$$

Now consider the limit of this ratio as Δt approaches 0, which is written as

$$f(t) = \lim_{\Delta t \to 0} \frac{F(t + \Delta t) - F(t)}{\Delta t} \tag{4}$$

Those who are familiar with calculus will recognize this limit, $f(t)$, as the derivative of $F(t)$ with respect to t, generally written $F'(t)$. This function is known as the *probability density function*, or simply the density function, of the random variable T. You might think of it as the instantaneous rate of change of the death probability with respect to time. Since $S(t) = 1 - F(t)$, it is not surprising that its instantaneous rate of change, $S'(t)$, is $-f(t) = -F'(t)$.

4.3 The Hazard Function

A third very useful way to characterize survival is by using a function called the *hazard function*, which we will usually denote by $h(t)$. It is the instantaneous rate of change of the death probability (as described in the previous section) conditioned on the patient's having survived to time t. The formula for the hazard is

$$h(t) = \frac{f(t)}{S(t)} = \frac{-S'(t)}{S(t)}, \ t \geq 0 \tag{5}$$

To understand why $f(t)$ is divided by $S(t)$, consider the probability of rolling a 3 on a toss of a six-sided die. Of course, that probability is 1/6. But suppose somebody tossed a die and told you that the result was an odd number. Then, what is the probability that the result is a 3, conditioned on the fact that the result is odd? Since there are now only three possible outcomes (1, 3, and 5) and all are equally likely, the answer is 1/3. That answer can be obtained by dividing 1/6 by 1/2, which is the probability of rolling an odd number. In the same manner, you can calculate the instantaneous change in the death probability at time t, conditioned on survival to time t, by dividing $f(t)$ by the probability of surviving to time t, $S(t)$.

Although the hazard at time t conveys information about the risk of death at that time for a patient who has survived for that long, you should not think of the hazard as a probability. In fact, it may exceed 1.0. A way to associate the hazard, $h(t)$, at time t, with a probability is to note that, based on equation 5 and the definition of $f(t)$, you can calculate the approximation for Δt near 0, of

$$h(t)\Delta t \doteq \frac{F(t + \Delta t) - F(t)}{S(t)} \tag{6}$$

The numerator in equation 6 is the probability that the patient dies by time $t + \Delta t$ minus the probability that he or she dies by time t; that is, the numerator is the probability that the patient dies at the time between t and $t + \Delta t$. As noted above, dividing by $S(t)$ conditions on surviving to time t. Thus the hazard at time t multiplied by a small increment of time approximates the probability of dying within that increment of time after t for a patient who survived to time t.

Using a fundamental theorem of calculus, if we plot the graph of the function $y = f(t)$, then for any value, t_0, of t, $F(t_0)$ is the area above the horizontal axis, under the curve, and to the left of a vertical line at t_0. $S(t_0)$ is the area to the right of t_0. Figure 1.3 illustrates this property for $t_0 = 3$ and an arbitrary density function $f(t)$.

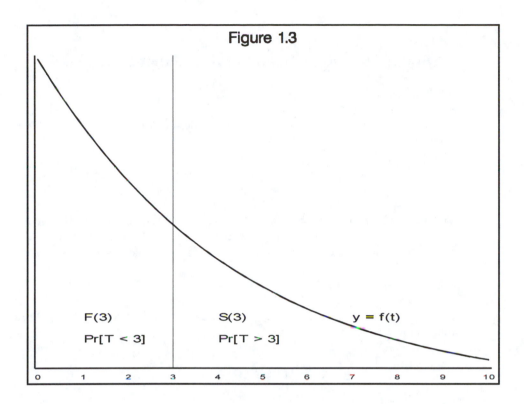

Figure 1.3

F(3)   S(3)   y = f(t)

Pr[T < 3]   Pr[T > 3]

0   1   2   3   4   5   6   7   8   9   10

Another important relationship between the functions that describe survival is given by

$$S(t) = \exp[-\int_0^t h(u)du] \tag{7}$$

The integral in equation 7 is called the cumulative hazard at time t, and it plays a critical role in long-term survival. If this integral increases without bound as $t \to \infty$, then $S(t)$ approaches 0 as $t \to \infty$. In other words, there are no long-term survivors or "cures." If, however, the integral approaches a limit, $c < \infty$, as $t \to \infty$, then $S(t)$ approaches exp(-c) as $t \to \infty$. In this case, we can think of exp(-c) as the *cure rate*. Estimation of a cure rate is one of the most important and challenging problems of survival analysis. An approach to this problem will be presented in Chapter 5.

5. Some Commonly Used Survival Functions

5.1 The Exponential Function

The simplest function that you can use to describe survival is the exponential function given by

$$S(t) \ = \ \exp(-\lambda t), \ t \geq 0 \tag{8}$$

This survival function has only one parameter, the constant hazard, λ. The median survival time, defined as the solution of $S(t) = 0.5$, is $t = -\log_e(0.5)/\lambda$. Also, if we assume a probability of p of surviving for time t, then λ is determined by $\lambda = -\log_e(p)/t$.

5.2 The Weibull Function

A more complex, but often more realistic, model for survival is given by the Weibull function

$$S(t) \ = \ \exp(-\lambda t^{\gamma}), \ t \geq 0 \tag{9}$$

Note that the exponential survival function is a special case of the Weibull function where $\gamma = 1$. The hazard function is given by $h(t) = \lambda \gamma t^{\gamma-1}$. It increases as t increases if $\gamma > 1$, and decreases as t increases if $0 < \gamma < 1$

Graphs of survival functions of each type are shown in Figures 1.4 and 1.5.

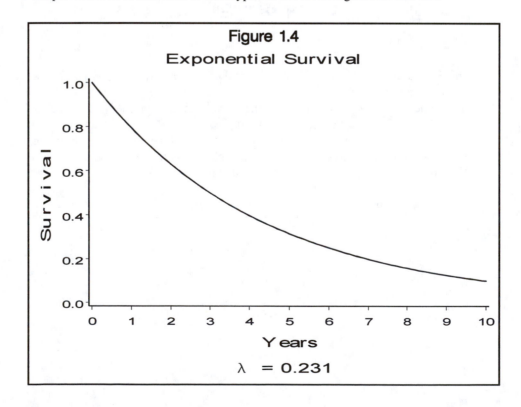

Figure 1.4

Exponential Survival

Years

$\lambda \ = \ 0.231$

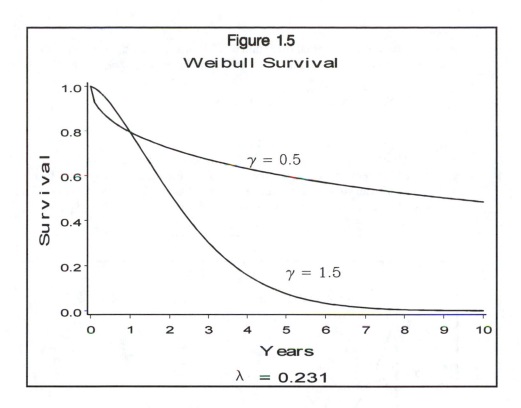

Figure 1.5
Weibull Survival

$\gamma = 0.5$

$\gamma = 1.5$

$\lambda = 0.231$

Other functions, such as the lognormal, gamma, and Rayleigh, are also sometimes used to describe survival, but will not be discussed in this chapter.

6. Functions that Allow for Cure

6.1 The Idea of *Cure Models*

The survival functions described in the previous section are all based on proper distribution functions, that is $F(t) \to 1$ as $t \to \infty$. Of course, this means that $S(t) \to 0$ as $t \to \infty$. Often, however, a model, to be realistic, must allow for a nonzero probability of indefinite survival – that is, a nonzero probability of cure. Suppose you were analyzing survival data for a cohort of children who had Hodgkin's Disease. You might find that a considerable number of patients were alive, apparently free of disease and still being followed after ten years, and that no deaths had occurred after four years. You could assume that a nonzero proportion had been cured in this case. A survival function that goes to zero with increasing time is not a good model for such data.

Figures 1.6, 1.7, and 1.8 graphically illustrate three types of survival functions that allow for cure. For purposes of comparison, the parameters in each case are chosen so that the cure rate is 30% and the noncures have a median survival time of one year.

6.2 Mixed Models

One way to model such data is to assume that the population being studied is a mixture of two subpopulations. A proportion, π, is cured, and the remaining proportion, $1-\pi$, has a survival function as described in section 6.1. If, for example, the survival function of the non-cured patients is exponential, the survival of the entire population can be given by

$$S(t) = \pi + (1 - \pi)\exp(-\lambda t), \ t \geq 0 \tag{10}$$

The graph of such a survival function approaches a plateau at $S(t) = \pi$ as $t \to \infty$. This model has been studied by Goldman (1984) and Sposto and Sather (1985). Figure 1.6 illustrates this example. Of course, the exponential function in equation 10 can be replaced by any survival function. For example, Gamel et al. (1994) have considered such a model based on a lognormal survival function for the non-cured patients.

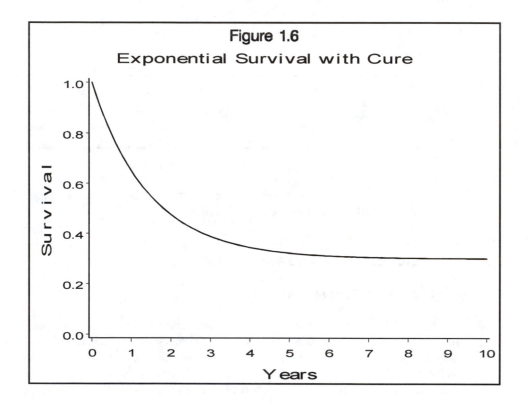

Figure 1.6
Exponential Survival with Cure

6.3 The Piecewise Exponential Model

Another model that can allow for cure is the piecewise exponential model as described by Shuster (1990). This model assumes that the hazard is constant over intervals, but can be different for different intervals. For example, we suppose that $h(t)=\lambda$ for $0 \le t < t_0$ and $h(t)=0$ for $t \ge t_0$. For this model, the survival function is given by

$$S(t) = \exp(-\lambda t) \; for \; 0 \le t < t_0$$
$$S(t) = \exp(-\lambda t_0) \; for \; t \ge t_0$$

(11)

Figure 1.7 illustrates this example.

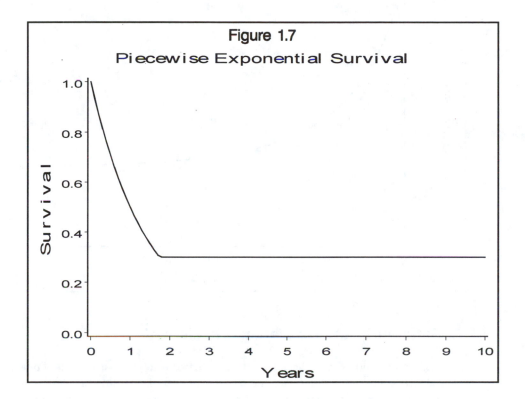

Figure 1.7
Piecewise Exponential Survival

6.4 The Gompertz Model

Still another model for survival that allows for cure is given by the Gompertz function, which is defined by

$$S(t) = \exp\{-\frac{\gamma}{\theta}[\exp(\theta t) - 1]\} \quad \gamma > 0, \, t \ge 0$$

(12)

Although this function appears to be rather complicated, it follows by equation 7 from the assumption that $h(t)$ is increasing or decreasing exponentially with rate θ as t increases. In fact, this function was first used by Gompertz (1825) to describe mortality in an aging male population in which he observed an exponentially increasing hazard. With $\theta < 0$, it's not hard to see that $S(t) \rightarrow \exp(\gamma/\theta)$ as $t \rightarrow \infty$. This function was first used to describe survival of patients by Haybittle (1959). It has also been studied in this context by others (Gehan and Siddiqui, 1973; Cantor and Shuster, 1990; and Garg, Rao, and Redmond, 1970). $S(t) \rightarrow \exp(-\gamma t)$ as $\theta \rightarrow 0$, so that the exponential function can be thought of as a special case of the Gompertz function with $\theta = 0$. Figure 1.8 illustrates this example.

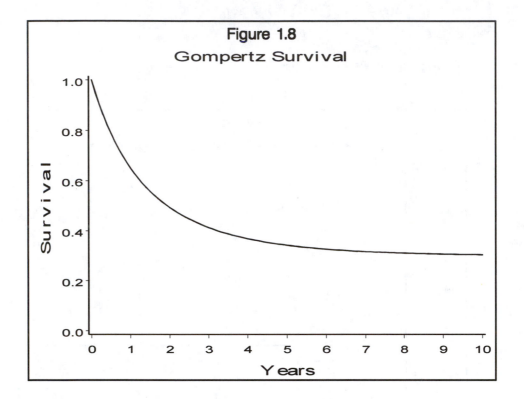

Figure 1.8

Gompertz Survival

7. Parametric and Nonparametric Methods

If you are willing to assume that survival can be described by a distribution of one of the types described in this chapter, then the way to use a set of sample data to make estimates or inferences about the underlying population is clear. You need to somehow obtain estimates of the parameter(s) that determine the distribution. Then, the desired estimates follow almost immediately. For example, assume that survival in a particular cohort can be described by the exponential model in equation 8. Then, if λ is estimated (by using methods to be described later in this book) to be 0.043 where the unit of time is years, then $\exp(-3 \times 0.043) = \exp(-0.129) = 0.879$ is the estimated probability of survival for at least three years. Furthermore, if the standard error of the estimate of λ is known, then standard methods permit us to calculate the standard error of the estimate of $S(t)$ and confidence intervals for $S(3)$. Similarly, if exponentiality is assumed for survival of patients in each of two treatment arms, then the superiority of one of the treatments is equivalent to its having a smaller λ. These matters will be discussed in more detail in Chapter 5.

Often, however, statisticians are reluctant to base analyses on assumed types of distributions. Many statistical methods, such as *t* tests and ANOVA, are rather robust to the assumption of normality for reasonably large sample sizes. Thus, inferences can often be made with some confidence even if you are not confident of normality. This is not true for methods of survival analysis. An estimate or inference based on the assumption of exponentiality might be grossly erroneous if that assumption does not hold. Thus, you would rather make statements that hold regardless of the underlying distribution. To enable us to make such statements, a class of methods has been developed that are valid without any distributional assumptions, or sometimes with only very modest distributional assumptions. Because of their power and, in many cases, their simplicity and intuitive appeal, these methods have come to dominate. Most SAS procedures that are used for survival analysis, and most of this book, is based upon such methods.

8. Parameters, Estimates, and the "hat" Notation

The parametric models described in sections 5 and 6 are each characterized by one or more parameters that are generally denoted by Greek letters. Their values, of course, are not known to us, but later in this book you learn about ways to estimate them. It is important that you keep in mind the distinction between parameters and their estimates. A *parameter* is an unknown and unknowable characteristic of a population. We study a sample drawn from a population in order to derive estimates of parameters. Sometimes these estimates also lead to hypothesis tests about the parameters. It is helpful to have a notation for estimates that reminds us of the parameter we are estimating. This book uses the name of a parameter with a "hat" ($\hat{\ }$) over it to represent an estimate for the parameter. For example, $\hat{\lambda}$ is the notation used for an estimate of λ. How to calculate $\hat{\lambda}$ from a sample is discussed in Chapters 4 and 5. Similarly, if survival time in a given population is described by a survival function $S(t)$, the notation $\hat{S}(t)$ will be used for estimates of $S(t)$. Methods of calculating $\hat{S}(t)$ from a sample are discussed in Chapters 2, 4, and 5.

9. Some Common Assumptions

In the analysis of survival data, we are frequently concerned about the effect of a variable on survival. The treatment to which a patient is assigned might be such a variable. Other variables might be demographic – age, race, or sex, for example. Still others might be associated with the patient's disease – cancer stage, number of blocked arteries, Karnofsky status, and so on. There are many ways in which a variable can impact on survival. Suppose a variable that is thought to impact on survival is observed, and let $h(t, x)$ be the hazard at time t for a patient with a value of x for that variable. The survival function has the proportional hazards property if, for some positive number, c, we have for all values of t and x

$$\frac{h(t, x + 1)}{h(t, x)} = c \tag{13}$$

According to this assumption, the effect of the variable is multiplicative on the hazard function. Then, whether the hazard is increasing, decreasing, or not affected by increasing values of the variable depends upon whether that constant multiple is less than, greater than, or equal to 1. Another possible assumption is that the effect of a variable might be to accelerate (or decelerate) mortality. Let $S_1(t)$ and $S_2(t)$ be the survival functions for two values of a variable. Often, this variable is the treatment a patient received, so that $S_1(t)$ and $S_2(t)$ are the survival functions for the two treatments. Then, for some positive number, b, you might have $S_1(t) = S_2(bt)$ for all nonnegative values of t. In other words, the probability of surviving to time t for one value of the variable is the same as the probability of surviving to time bt for the other. This is called the *accelerated failure time assumption*. Whether the value associated with $S_1(t)$ is better than, worse than, or equivalent to the value associated with $S_2(t)$ depends upon whether b is less than, greater than, or equal to 1. While there are statistical methods that do not require such assumptions, as you shall see later in this book, often these assumptions are reasonable and can lead to more powerful and informative analyses. Assumptions such as these, which attribute certain properties to the underlying survival distribution without specifying its form, are said to be semiparametric. Methods based on such assumptions occupy a place between the nonparametric and parametric methods.

Chapter 2   Nonparametric Survival Function Estimation

1. The Kaplan-Meier Estimate of the Survival Function

In this chapter, the estimation of a survival function, $S(t)$, for various values of t from data of the form $(t_1, d_1), \ldots, (t_n, d_n)$ as described previously is discussed. For now, assume that the times are ordered so that $t_1 < t_2 < \ldots < t_n$. In Chapter 5, "Parametric Methods," you will learn about estimation methods that assume a survival distribution of a given form, but for now no such assumptions will be made.

1.1 An Example

Suppose that you follow ten patients for survival, and you observe the following times (in months):

5, 12, 25, 26, 27, 28, 37, 39, 40+, 42+

You would like to estimate the 36-month survival rate, that is, $S(36)$, from these data. Since four of the ten survived more than 36 months, it is reasonable to estimate $S(36)$, the probability of surviving at least 36 months by 4/10 or 0.40. Now suppose, however, that an additional three patients were censored at 32, 33, and 34 months respectively. Now the data look like this:

5, 12, 25, 26, 27, 28, 32+, 33+, 34+, 37, 39, 40+, 42+

What do you do now? On the one hand, you don't know whether any of these patients with censored times survived more than 36 months, so you might be inclined to omit them and still estimate $S(36)$ by 0.40. On the other hand, these three patients, known to have survived for more than 32, 33, and 34 months respectively, had better prospects of surviving at least 36 months than a patient who just entered. The problem is how to take the censored times 32+, 33+, and 34+ into consideration. The method that is discussed below, first presented by Kaplan and Meier (1958), allows you to correctly make use of such censored data in estimating $S(t)$.

Consider the above data. Because the first death occurs at 5 months, it is reasonable to estimate $S(t)$ by 1.00 for $0 \leq t < 5$. Of the 13 patients at risk just prior to 5 months, 12 survived past that time. Thus, you would estimate $S(t)$ by 12/13 for $t = 5$ or slightly more than 5. There's no reason to reduce that estimate prior to 12 months because there are no additional deaths until $t = 12$. Now, 11 of the 12 patients who survived past $t = 5$ survived past $t = 12$. Thus, the probability of surviving past 12 months, for those who survived past 5 months, is estimated to be 11/12. In order to survive past $t = 12$, one must first survive past $t = 5$ and then survive from $t = 5$ past $t = 12$. The probability of doing both is the product of the probabilities of each and is, therefore, estimated by (12/13)(11/12). Continuing in this fashion, the probability of surviving past 25 is estimated by (12/13)(11/12)(10/11), and the probability of surviving past 28 is estimated by (12/13)(11/12)(10/11)(9/10)(8/9)(7/8). Here is where the censored times play a role. The next death is at $t = 37$. But, because of the three censored times that occurred at times prior to 37, only four patients were at risk at $t = 37$. Three of them survived past 37 months. So you should estimate the probability of surviving past 37 months for those surviving past 28 months to be 3/4. The probability of surviving past 37 months is, therefore, estimated by (12/13)(11/12)(10/11)(9/10)(8/9)(7/8)(3/4).

Do you see the pattern in this? At each death time t_i, the probability of surviving past $t = t_i$ is reduced by being multiplied by $(r_i - 1)/r_i$ where r_i is the number at risk just prior to the i'th time. Censored times do not alter that probability, but they reduce the number at risk at succeeding death times. The above calculations for the estimated values of $S(t)$, denoted $\hat{S}(t)$, are illustrated in Table 2.1 below.

Table 2.1

i	t_i	d_i	r_i	$\hat{S}(t)\ t_i \leq t < t_{i+1}$
0	0	-	-	1.00
1	5	1	13	$12/13 = 0.92$
2	12	1	12	$0.92(11/12) = 0.85$
3	25	1	11	$0.85(10/110) = 0.77$
4	26	1	10	$0.77(9/10) = 0.69$
5	27	1	9	$0.69(8/9) = 0.62$
6	28	1	8	$0.62(7/8) = 0.54$
7	32	0	7	0.54
8	33	0	6	0.54
9	34	0	5	0.54
10	37	1	4	$0.54(3/4) = 0.40$
11	39	1	3	$0.40(2/3) = 0.27$
12	40	0	2	0.27
13	42	0	1	0.27

The above table is called a Kaplan-Meier, or product-limit, life table. In this table, each r_i is the number of patients at risk at time t_i, i.e. the number whose times are greater than or equal to t_i. Each d_i is 0 or 1, depending upon whether the time is a censored or a death time. The graphical representation of the calculated survival probabilities (shown in Figure 2.1) is often called a Kaplan-Meier survival curve. The estimates, $\hat{S}(t)$, are called Kaplan-Meier survival estimates.

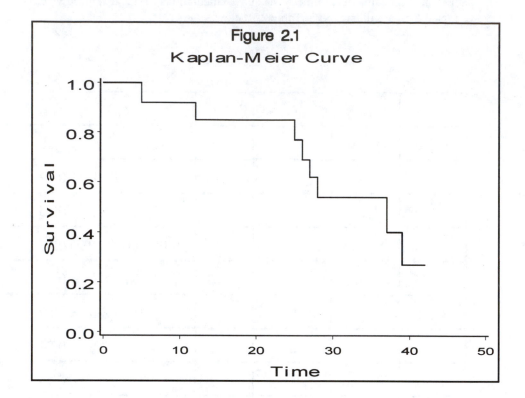

1.2 The Kaplan-Meier Estimation Formula

While, in theory, observation times should not contain ties, in actual practice ties are possible. This can be accounted for by letting the t_i be the observation times and, for any i, allowing for the possibility that there is more than one patient whose observation time is t_i. Let d_i be the number of deaths at time t_i. Then if there is only one patient whose time is t_i, this corresponds to the previous notation.

Examination of the above table should enable the reader to confirm the formula below:

$$\hat{S}(t) = \prod_{t_i \leq t} \left[\frac{r_i - d_i}{r_i} \right] \tag{1}$$

The popularity of the Kaplan-Meier method is due to several desirable properties possessed by the resultant estimator of $S(t)$. The most important is that, under rather mild assumptions regarding the censoring distribution, $\hat{S}(t)$ is asymptotically normally distributed with mean $S(t)$. This means that as the sample size gets larger and larger, the random variable, $\hat{S}(t)$, gets close to having a normal distribution. The mean value of that distribution is the true, unknown value of $S(t)$. Thus by calculating an estimate of the variance of $\hat{S}(t_0)$, we can construct confidence intervals for $S(t_0)$ and perform hypothesis tests concerning it. This is explored more fully later in this chapter.

2. The Actuarial Life Table

Long before the now-classic Kaplan and Meier paper, demographers and actuaries were using a method called the actuarial life table to study the longevity of natural populations. Although they were concerned with problems of predicting mortality rates in natural populations–rather than the survivorship of patients with a disease or subject to a particular treatment regimen–their methods can be applied to these situations as well. The actuarial life table is particularly suitable when, instead of knowing the actual survival and censoring times, you know only that they are in particular time intervals, such as the 0 to 3 months, 3 months to 6 months, etc.

2.1 The Actuarial Estimates

To construct the actuarial life table, start by partitioning the time axis into subintervals by the numbers $0 = \tau_0 < \tau_1 < \tau_2 < \ldots$ etc. The partitions are usually taken to be of equal length (for example, three months, six months, or one year), but that is not necessary. Suppose at time 0 we have N individuals at risk. Suppose that during the first interval, $[\tau_0, \tau_1)$, there are c_1 individuals censored. Then, the number of patients at risk during that interval went from N at time τ_0 to $N - c_1$ at time τ_1. It is reasonable to assume that it would not be introducing much error to consider the number at risk during this interval to be the average of these two values, $N - c_1/2$. This is called *the effective number at risk* in this interval. Since e_1 died in this interval, the probability of surviving through this interval is estimated to be $p_1 = 1 - e_1/(N - c_1/2)$. More generally, if r_i represents the number at risk at the beginning of the i'th interval, e_i represents the number who die in this interval, and c_i represents the number censored in this interval, then $r_i - c_i/2$ is thought of as the average (or effective) number at risk in the i'th interval, and $p_i = 1 - e_i/(r_i - c_i/2)$ is the estimated probability of surviving the i'th interval for those surviving all previous intervals. This is called the conditional survival for that interval. $S(\tau_i)$ would then be estimated by the product of the p_j's for $j \leq i$. The actuarial method is somewhat dependent on the choice of the τ_i's. It is sometimes preferred when the sample size and the number of deaths is quite large. In that case the Kaplan-Meier life table can be lengthy, while the actuarial table is more compact. In medical research, the Kaplan-

Meier method is generally preferred, and discussions that follow focus on that method. The actuarial life table for the data presented earlier in this chapter is shown in Table 2.2. A graph of this estimated survival function produced by this method is given as Figure 2.2. Interval widths were chosen to be six months, although other choices are possible.

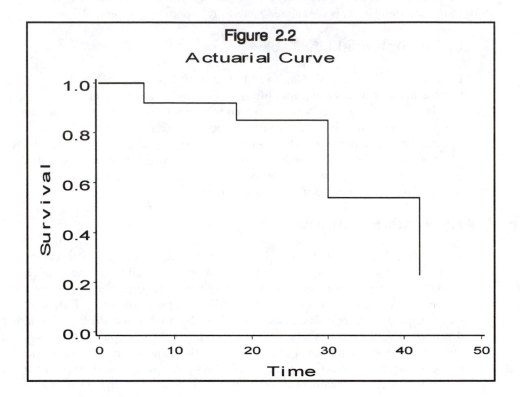

Table 2.2

Interval (months)	Number Entering Interval	Number Censored	Effective Number in Interval	Deaths in Interval	Conditional Survival	Cumulative Survival
[0, 6)	13	0	13.0	1	0.92	1.00
[6, 12)	12	0	12.0	0	1.00	0.92
[12, 18)	12	0	12.0	1	1.00	0.92
[18, 24)	11	0	11.0	0	1.00	0.85
[24, 30)	11	0	11.0	4	0.64	0.85
[30, 36)	7	3	5.5	0	1.00	0.54
[36, 42)	4	1	3.5	2	0.43	0.54
[42, 4)	1	1	0.5	0	1.00	0.23

2.2 Estimates of Other Functions

The actuarial method is also called the life table method in the documentation for PROC LIFETEST. This method can also produce estimates of the density and hazard functions at the midpoint of each subinterval. Approximating the derivative in formula 4 of Chapter 1 by a fraction used in defining that derivative, you can estimate the density $f(t_{mi})$ by

$$\hat{f}(\tau_{m_i}) = [\hat{S}_a(\tau_{i-1}) - \hat{S}_a(\tau_i)] / (\tau_i - \tau_{i-1}) \tag{2}$$

where τ_{mi} is the midpoint of the i'th subinterval and $\hat{S}_a(.)$ represents actuarial survival estimates. Furthermore, we can estimate the hazard $h(t_{mi})$ by $\hat{h}(t_{mi}) = \hat{f}(\tau_{mi})/\hat{S}_a(\tau_{mi})$ where $\hat{S}_a(\tau_{mi})$ is estimated by $[\hat{S}_a(\tau_{i-1}) + \hat{S}_a(\tau_i)]/2$. A little algebra shows that this hazard estimate for the midpoint of the interval $(\tau_{i-1} - \tau_i)$ can be written as

$$\hat{h}(\tau_{m_i}) = e_i/\{[r_i - (c_i + e_i)/2)](\tau_i - \tau_{i-1})\} \tag{3}$$

Note that this estimate can be thought of as the estimated probability of dying in an interval in which there were e_i deaths and an "average" of $r_i - (c_i + e_i)/2$ at risk divided by the length of the interval. These estimates may not be very good for small samples.

3. Estimates of the Variance of the Kaplan-Meier Estimator

3.1 Greenwood's Formula

Two formulas have been advocated and used for estimating the variance of the Kaplan-Meier estimate of the survival function. The most popular one is Greenwood's formula (Greenwood 1926). It is the method used by PROC LIFETEST. Greenwood's formula is given by

$$var[\hat{S}(t)] \approx [\hat{S}(t)]^2 \sum_{t_i \leq t} \frac{d_i}{r_i(r_i - d_i)} \tag{4}$$

The mathematical derivation of this formula is discussed at the end of this chapter. Note that times at which patients are censored (that is, $d_i = 0$) do not increase this variance estimate, although estimates of $S(t)$ for times past t_i are based on fewer patients. Thus, the above formula may understate, sometimes quite drastically, the true variance of $\hat{S}(t)$.

3.2 Peto's Formula

Another formula that has been proposed is Peto's formula (Peto et al. 1977). Let $R(t)$ be the number of patients at risk at time t. That is, $R(t)$ is the number of patients who have not died or been censored with times less than t. Peto's formula is given by

$$var[\hat{S}(t)] \approx \frac{[\hat{S}(t)]^2[1 - \hat{S}(t)]}{R(t)} \tag{5}$$

The justification for this formula for estimating the variance of $\hat{S}(t)$ is quite simple. If no patients had censored times less than t, then $\hat{S}(t)$ would be an estimate of a binomial proportion, and its variance would be $\hat{S}(t)[1 - \hat{S}(t)]/N$ where N is the number of patients in the study. In that case, $R(t) = N\hat{S}(t)$ and formula 5 is exact. If some patients are censored at times less than t, then $R(t) < N\hat{S}(t)$. Thus formula 5 overestimates the variance, but, it is claimed, not by much. Also, note that formula 5 produces variance estimates that are increased as the number at risk is diminished either by death or censoring. Finally, note that formula 5 can be used to predict the variance of a Kaplan-Meier estimate at a given time for a study that has yet to be performed. This may be important when a study is being planned. When planning a study whose main objective is to estimate the survival function for patients undergoing a certain treatment, you might want to make sure that a Kaplan-Meier estimate, say for three-year survival, has reasonable precision; that is, it has small variance. You will see later in this chapter how to choose a sample size that ensures that the Peto estimate of the variance is sufficiently small.

4. Hypothesis Tests and Confidence Intervals Based on Asymptotic Normality

4.1 Hypothesis Tests

From the fact that $\hat{S}(t)$ is asymptotically normal with mean $S(t)$, we can take $\hat{S}(t)/[\text{var}(\hat{S}(t)]^{1/2}$ to be distributed, approximately, as a standard normal random variable for reasonably large sample sizes. This, in turn, leads to hypothesis tests involving $S(t)$. For example, for a specific value, t_0, of t, we would reject the null hypothesis of H_0: $S(t_0) = p$ in favor of the alternative H_A: $S(t_0) \neq p$ at the 0.05 significance level if and only if $|\hat{S}(t_0) - p| \geq 1.96\{\text{var}[\hat{S}(t_0)]\}^{1/2}$. Also, if $S_1(t)$ and $S_2(t)$ are survival functions for two independent groups and $\hat{S}_1(t)$ and $\hat{S}_2(t)$ are their Kaplan-Meier estimates then, for any value t_0 of t, we would reject the null hypothesis H_0: $S_1(t_0) = S_2(t_0)$ in favor of the alternative H_A: $S_1(t_0) \neq S_2(t_0)$ at the 0.05 significance level if and only if $|\hat{S}_1(t_0) - \hat{S}_2(t_0)| \geq 1.96\{\text{var}[\hat{S}_1(t_0)] + \text{var}[\hat{S}_2(t_0)]\}^{1/2}$. Generally, however, it is preferable to compare survival curves using methods, such as those to be introduced in the next chapter, which take the entire survival curves into consideration.

4.2 Confidence Intervals

We can, of course, write a $(1-\alpha)100\%$ confidence interval for $S(t_0)$ as $\hat{S}(t_0) \pm z_{\alpha/2}\{\text{var}[\hat{S}(t_0)]\}^{1/2}$. A problem with this approach is that it sometimes leads to confidence limits outside the permissible range (0 to 1) of $S(t)$. One solution to this is to simply replace any computed limit that is out of this range by 0 or 1. Kalbfleisch and Prentice (1980) suggest, as another approach, that approximate upper and lower confidence bounds are given by the expression $\hat{S}(t)^{\exp(\pm x)}$ where x is given by

$$ x = \frac{z_{\alpha/2}}{\hat{S}(t)\log_e \hat{S}(t)}\sqrt{var[\hat{S}(t)]} \tag{6} $$

The endpoints of any such interval are always between 0 and 1. In formula 6, either the Greenwood or Peto formula can be used for $\text{var}[\hat{S}(t)]$. The latter gives more conservative (wider) confidence intervals. The justification for this result is given at the end of this chapter. *The reader should keep in mind that both confidence interval methods refer to pointwise confidence intervals for specified values, t_0, of t.* That is, for a value of t, values of random variables L and U are calculated such that the interval (L, U) has a probability of $(1-\alpha)100\%$ of containing $S(t)$. This is not the same as constructing functions $L(t)$ and $U(t)$ such that the probability that $L(t) < S(t) < U(t)$ for all values of t is $(1-\alpha)100\%$. Such a pair of functions define what are often called $(1-\alpha)100\%$ confidence bands for $S(t)$. While such techniques have been described, by Hall and Wellner (1980) for example, they will not be discussed here.

5. Some Problems with the Kaplan-Meier Estimator of S(t)

There are other nonparametric estimators of $S(t)$. Nelson (1969), Reid (1981), and Sander (1975) have proposed alternatives, but none has approached the popularity of the Kaplan-

Meier estimator. Thus they will not be discussed further here. We should, however, point out some shortcomings of the Kaplan-Meier estimator. One problem, discussed in detail by Miller (1983), is the low efficiency of the estimates relative to the estimators that are associated with parametric models. That is, for a given sample, the variance of $\hat{S}(t)$ will be greater than the corresponding variance of the estimator based on a parametric model. This problem is most severe for larger values of t – precisely those values we are likely to be most interested in. Another problem with the Kaplan-Meier estimator is the counter-intuitive property that later deaths tend to lower the estimated survival curve more than earlier deaths. This phenomenon has been reported and described by Cantor and Shuster (1992) and by Oakes (1993), although it probably has been noticed by others as well. To see how this happens, consider the set of survival data given as an example in the first section of this chapter. Now suppose you learn that the death that was recorded as happening at $t = 5$ actually did not occur until $t = 41$. This will change the Kaplan-Meier life table. It will now be as Table 2.3.

Table 2.3

i	t_i	d_i	r_i	$\hat{S}(t)\ t_i \le t < t_{i+1}$
0	0	-	-	1.00
1	12	1	13	12/13 = 0.92
2	25	1	12	0.92(11/12) = 0.85
3	26	1	11	0.85(10/110 = 0.77
4	27	1	10	0.77(9/10) = 0.69
5	28	1	9	0.69(7/8) = 0.62
6	32	0	8	0.62
7	33	0	7	0.62
8	34	0	6	0.62
9	37	1	5	0.62(4/5) = 0.49
10	39	1	4	0.49(3/4) = 0.37
11	40	0	3	0.37
12	41	1	2	0.37(1/2) = 18
13	42	0	1	0.18

Compare this table to the table in the first section. In the "right hand tail," the revised table actually has smaller estimated survival probabilities. Because later survival probabilities tend to be of greater interest, the revised table, with everything the same except that one death had a later time, indicate worse survival. This seems to contradict the fact that the revised data, with one death delayed from 5 months to 41 months, apparently indicates better survival. Closer scrutiny of the calculations shows how this happened arithmetically. In the earlier table, the death at time $t = 5$, when there were 13 patients at risk, diminished the survival probability by a factor of 12/13. In the later table, this factor no longer appears, but the death when there were only two patients at risk reduces the survival probability by a factor of 1/2. An even more extreme example would be created if the patient who had been observed longest had died. In that case, the final survival probability estimate would be zero. This is not simply an arithmetical oddity that rarely occurs. Consider a study in which patients with cancer are followed for both disease free survival and survival. An event for the disease-free survival analysis would be death from any cause, or recurrence of tumor. By definition, the true survival curve for disease free survival must be below the corresponding curve for survival. After all, for any time t, one has greater probability of dying or having disease recurrence by time t than of dying by that time. If, however, patients tend to die after their tumors recur, then, as in the above example, the Kaplan-Meier survival curve for survival can be below the Kaplan-Meier curve for disease-free survival.

6 Using PROC LIFETEST

6.1 Introduction to PROC LIFETEST

PROC LIFETEST produces Kaplan-Meier and actuarial life tables and graphs. Specifically, this procedure produces output that includes the survival distribution estimates as well as the Greenwood estimate of their standard errors. It can also produce comparisons of survival distributions, but this is discussed in the next chapter. To use this procedure, you must have a SAS data set with a time variable. Generally you will have a variable that indicates whether or not the time is complete or censored also, although that is not neccesary if no times are censored. In this book, this variable is taken to have the values 0 and 1, depending on whether the time is censored or complete, respectively. PROC LIFETEST does not require that these values be used. You can specify any set of values that can indicate that the time is censored. This is true of the macros that are introduced later as well. This can be handy if the data contain values that indicate different reasons for censoring.

6.2 Syntax for PROC LIFETEST

The basic for syntax for PROC LIFETEST looks like this:

```
proc lifetest <options>;
time   timevar<*eventvar(list of values)>;
```

Here, *timevar* is the name of the variable that gives the amount of time a patient was followed, and *eventvar* is the name of the variable that tells whether or not the event was observed. If there are no censored times, then you can specify the time statement with only the time variable. The list in parentheses gives the values that indicate the time is censored. As with other SAS procedures, the data set to be used is taken to be the last one created if it is not specified in the invocation of the procedure. Of course, as with many other SAS procedures, PROC LIFETEST can do analyses for distinct subgroups of the sample with a BY statement, and you can use the subsetting WHERE to restrict the analysis to a subset of the data. The following is a list of the most common options that you might want to use. Many other options can be found in the SAS documentation for the LIFETEST procedure.

- PLOTS = (*list*) produces graphs of some useful functions. The words in *list* can be chosen from

  SURVIVAL or S   for a graph of the estimated survival function versus time

  HAZARD or H   for a graph of the hazard function versus time

  PDF or P   for a graph of the density function versus time

  LOGSURV or LS   for a graph of $\log_e \hat{S}(t)$ versus time

  LOGLOGS or LLS   for a graph of $\log_e[-\log_e \hat{S}(t)]$ versus $\log_e(t)$

  The request for the hazard and density graphs are valid only if the actuarial method is used. The graphs of $\log_e \hat{S}(t)$ versus time and $\log_e[-\log_e \hat{S}(t)]$ versus $\log_e(t)$ can be helpful in deciding on a parametric model. This will be discussed in Chapter 5.

- METHOD = *type* specifies the type of survival estimate calculated. Using PL or KM for *type* produces Kaplan-Meier estimates. (PL stands for "*product-limit*", another name for the Kaplan-Meier estimate.) Specifying ACT or LIFE or LT produces actuarial estimates. If the METHOD= option is not used, Kaplan-Meier estimates are produced by default. If the actuarial method is chosen, the output includes hazard and density function estimates at the interval midpoints as well as their standard errors.

- If you choose actuarial estimates, you can specify the intervals used in several ways. You can give the endpoints explicitly by a statement like INTERVALS = 2, 4, 6, 8, 10, 12 or INTERVALS = 2 TO 12 BY 2. Note that the first interval will start with 0 even if that value is not given. Instead, you can specify the width of each interval with a statement of the form WIDTH = *value*. A third choice is to specify the number of intervals with a statement of the form NINTERVAL = *value*. PROC LIFETEST will then divide the entire range of times by the number chosen. It may alter that number slightly to produce endpoints that are round numbers. Finally, you can use none of these choices. In that case, PROC LIFETEST will proceed as if NINTERVAL = 10 was specified.

- If you want to produce not only output, but also a SAS data set which contains the survival function estimates as well as lower and upper bounds for a confidence interval for the survival function, you can specify OUTSURV = *dataset-name* or OUTS = *dataset-name*. You might want to do this in order to use the values in this data set for further calculations or analyses. If the actuarial method is used, you also get confidence intervals for the density function and hazard function. The default is to get 95% confidence intervals. You can override that with the option ALPHA = *value*. This will produce $(1 - value)100\%$ confidence intervals. Note that the confidence intervals are symmetric of the form estimator $\pm z_{\alpha/2}se$. For the survival estimate confidence interval, *se* is the square root of the Greenwood variance, and bounds below 0.0 or above 1.0 are replaced by 0.0 and 1.0, respectively.

Starting with Release 6.07.03, you can specify GRAPHICS as an option. This causes any plots requested to be produced in high resolution. The GRAPHICS option is valid only if you license SAS/GRAPH software. If you use this option, it is recommended that you first use a GOPTIONS statement and a SYMBOL statement. In Releases 6.07.03 through 6.09, there is a "bug" in this option. Graphs are extended to the right as far as the right-hand boundary of the coordinate system, even if this is beyond the data. SAS Note 9667 shows how to circumvent this "bug," which was fixed in Release 6.10.

Starting with Release 6.11, you can use an option of the form TIMELIST = *list*, where *list* is a list of time values. This option can be used to produce a Kaplan-Meier table that contains rows for only those times in the list. By using this option, you can produce more compact printouts. For example, suppose you have survival data for 500 patients with follow-up of up to 10 years. Without this option the Kaplan-Meier life table could contain up to 500 lines, one for each distinct time. If you use the option TIMELIST = 1 2 3 4 5 6 7 8 9 10, you would produce a lifetable with only 10 lines.

7. An Example of the Use of PROC LIFETEST

Example 2.1 shows how PROC LIFETEST can be used. This example uses data generated in a clinical trial for the treatment of pediatric leukemia that was conducted by the Southwest Oncology Group. The event of interest was death and the time is in years. The data from this study continue to be maintained by the Pediatric Oncology Group, which graciously provided, through its statistician, Jonathan Shuster, permission for its use. Output 2.1 shows the results.

Example 2.1

```
data;
        input time d @@;
        cards;
0.0493 1    0.2849 1    0.4082 1    0.8767 1    0.8877 1    1.1233 1
1.2247 0    1.3753 1    1.5425 1    1.5836 1    1.7397 1    1.7589 1
1.7726 1    1.9233 1    1.9562 0    2.0493 1    2.2986 1    2.3425 1
3.7315 1    4.0548 1    4.0685 0    4.5863 1    4.9534 1    5.1534 0
5.7315 0    5.8493 1    5.8685 1    6.0712 0    6.1151 0    7.3781 0
7.6630 0    8.0438 0    8.1890 0    8.2055 0    8.2548 0    8.4274 0
8.4521 0    8.7589 0    9.0356 0    9.8959 0    9.9151 0    9.9178 0
10.1151 0   10.4027 0   10.6000 0   10.6603 1   10.6685 0   10.7260 0
10.9260 0   10.9370 0   11.2027 0   11.4548 0   11.4712 0   11.5589 0
11.6082 0   11.6164 0   11.6521 0   11.7123 0   11.7671 0   11.8466 0
11.8575 0   11.8685 0   11.9863 0   12.0082 0
;

proc lifetest plots=(s);
        time time*d(0);
run;
```

Output 2.1

The LIFETEST Procedure

Product-Limit Survival Estimates

TIME	Survival	Failure	Survival Standard Error	Number Failed	Number Left
0.0000	1.0000	0	0	0	64
0.0493	0.9844	0.0156	0.0155	1	63
0.2849	0.9688	0.0313	0.0217	2	62
0.4082	0.9531	0.0469	0.0264	3	61
0.8767	0.9375	0.0625	0.0303	4	60
0.8877	0.9219	0.0781	0.0335	5	59
1.1233	0.9063	0.0938	0.0364	6	58
1.2247*	.	.	.	6	57
1.3753	0.8904	0.1096	0.0391	7	56
1.5425	0.8745	0.1255	0.0415	8	55
1.5836	0.8586	0.1414	0.0437	9	54
1.7397	0.8427	0.1573	0.0457	10	53
1.7589	0.8268	0.1732	0.0475	11	52
1.7726	0.8109	0.1891	0.0492	12	51
1.9233	0.7950	0.2050	0.0507	13	50
1.9562*	.	.	.	13	49
2.0493	0.7787	0.2213	0.0522	14	48
2.2986	0.7625	0.2375	0.0536	15	47
2.3425	0.7463	0.2537	0.0549	16	46
3.7315	0.7301	0.2699	0.0560	17	45
4.0548	0.7138	0.2862	0.0571	18	44
4.0685*	.	.	.	18	43
4.5863	0.6972	0.3028	0.0581	19	42
4.9534	0.6806	0.3194	0.0590	20	41
5.1534*	.	.	.	20	40
5.7315*	.	.	.	20	39
5.8493	0.6632	0.3368	0.0601	21	38
5.8685	0.6457	0.3543	0.0610	22	37
6.0712*	.	.	.	22	36
6.1151*	.	.	.	22	35
7.3781*	.	.	.	22	34
7.6630*	.	.	.	22	33
8.0438*	.	.	.	22	32
8.1890*	.	.	.	22	31
8.2055*	.	.	.	22	30
8.2548*	.	.	.	22	29
8.4274*	.	.	.	22	28
8.4521*	.	.	.	22	27
8.7589*	.	.	.	22	26
9.0356*	.	.	.	22	25
9.8959*	.	.	.	22	24
9.9151*	.	.	.	22	23
9.9178*	.	.	.	22	22
10.1151*	.	.	.	22	21
10.4027*	.	.	.	22	20

10.6000*	.	.	.	22	19
10.6603	0.6117	0.3883	0.0666	23	18
10.6685*	.	.	.	23	17
10.7260*	.	.	.	23	16
10.9260*	.	.	.	23	15
10.9370*	.	.	.	23	14
11.2027*	.	.	.	23	13
11.4548*	.	.	.	23	12
11.4712*	.	.	.	23	11
11.5589*	.	.	.	23	10
11.6082*	.	.	.	23	9
11.6164*	.	.	.	23	8
11.6521*	.	.	.	23	7
11.7123*	.	.	.	23	6
11.7671*	.	.	.	23	5
11.8466*	.	.	.	23	4
11.8575*	.	.	.	23	3
11.8685*	.	.	.	23	2
11.9863*	.	.	.	23	1
12.0082*	.	.	.	23	0

* Censored Observation

The LIFETEST Procedure

Summary Statistics for Time Variable TIME

Quantile	Point Estimate	95% Confidence Interval [Lower, Upper)	
75%	.	.	.
50%	.	10.6603	.
25%	2.3425	1.7589	10.6603

Mean   7.7241   Standard Error   0.5297

NOTE: The last observation was censored so the estimate of the mean is biased.

Summary of the Number of Censored and Uncensored Values

Total	Failed	Censored	%Censored
64	23	41	64.0625

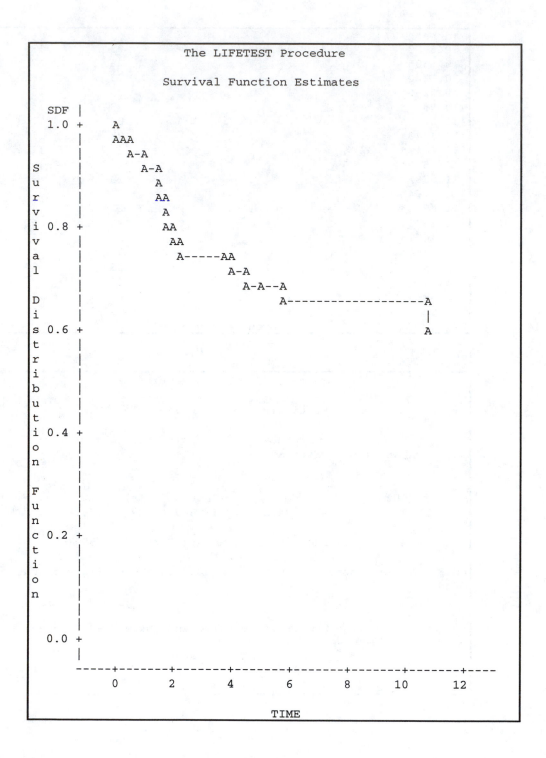

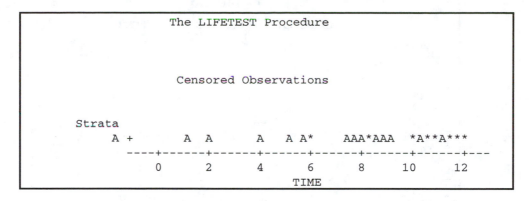

Note that the output does not give values of the estimated survival function or the standard error for censored survival times. They should be taken to be the values associated with the preceding complete observation. In fact, if t_i and t_j are consecutive complete times, then we would take $\hat{S}(t) = \hat{S}(t_i)$ and $\mathrm{var}[\hat{S}(t)] = \mathrm{var}[\hat{S}(t_i)]$ for $t_i \le t < t_j$. Also note that the survival curve ends with the last complete observation at $t = 10.6603$. Many analysts would continue the curve with a horizontal line to the last censored time. In addition to the life table, PROC LIFETEST also gives an estimate of the mean survival time and the quartiles of the survival distribution, if defined. The estimated mean survival time is simply the area under the Kaplan-Meier survival curve to the left of the largest event time. This estimate is biased in the direction of being too low if the largest time is censored. The estimate, 2.3425, given above for the 25th percentile, means that $t = 2.3425$ is the estimated time that it would take for 25% to die (or experience the event being studied). The 50th percentile (or median) and 75th percentile are similarly defined. In the example above, no 50th or 75th percentiles are given because the final survival estimate exceeded 50%. The one-dimensional graph of the censored times is particularly useful if two or more groups are being compared. In that situation, this graph may indicate that patients are quitting the study or otherwise being lost to follow-up differentially. This might require further inquiries. If the GRAPHICS option is used in the PROC LIFETEST statement, then the high-resolution graph shown as Figure 2.3 will replace the survival curve above.

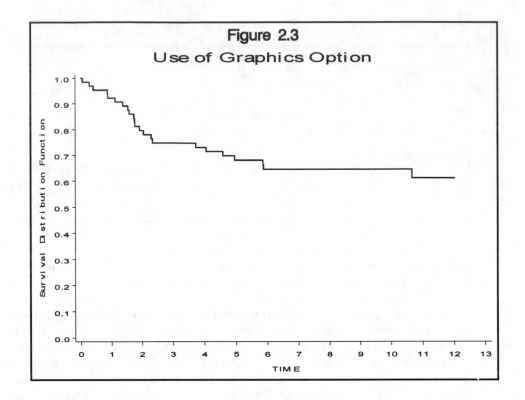

8. Two Macros as Alternatives to PROC LIFETEST

This section describes two macros that offer some features not available in PROC LIFETEST. The first is the macro KMTABLE. It gives you the option of specifying either the Greenwood or Peto formula for the variance of $\hat{S}(t)$ and either $\hat{S}(t) \pm z_{\alpha/2}[\text{var}\hat{S}(t)]^{1/2}$ or formula 6 for $(1-\alpha)100\%$ confidence intervals. The macro KMTABLE, is given at the end of this chapter.

The template below facilitates the use of this macro. You can simply insert it into your program after you have included a file containing the macro KMTABLE and have defined the data set to be used.

```
%kmtable(
          dataset=          /* default is _last_ */
          ,pct=             /* default is 95 for 95% CI */
          ,time=            /* time variable */
          ,cens=            /* variable indicating censored
                               or complete times */
          ,censval=         /* value(s) that indicate censored
                               observation */
          ,method=          /* 1 for method used in Proc Lifetest
                               2 for method that yields limits in
                               (0,1) */
          ,variance=        /* G or g for Greenwood's formula, P or
                               p for Peto's formula */
          ,byvar=           /* optional variable for separate
                               tables */
          ,print=           /* yes (default) to print table, no to
                               suppress printing */
          )
```

As an example of the use of this macro, consider the data set to which we applied PROC LIFETEST earlier in this chapter.

After defining this data set, you can simply insert the above template with the parameters filled in as in Example 2.2

Example 2.2

```
%kmtable(
          dataset= leuk    /* default is _last_ */
                           /* default is 95 for 95% CI */
          ,time= time      /* time variable */
          ,cens=d          /* variable indicating censored
                              or complete times */
          ,censval= 0      /* value(s) that indicate censored
                              observation */
          ,method= 2       /* 1 for method used in Proc Lifetest
                              2 for method that yields limits in
                              (0,1) */
          ,variance=p      /* G or g for Greenwood's formula, P or
                              p for Peto's formula */
                           /* optional variable for separate
                              tables   */
                           /* yes (default) to print table, no to
                              suppress printing */
          )
```

or equivalently

```
%kmtable(dataset=leuk, time=time, cens=d, censval=0, method=2,
         variance=p)
```

This invocation of the macro KMTABLE produces Output 2.2

Output 2.2

| | | | The SAS System | | | |

OBS	TIME	D	Survival Distribution Function Estimate	Peto stderr	Method 2 95 pct lcl	Method 2 95 pct ucl
1	0.0000	1	1.00000	0.00000	1.00000	1.00000
2	0.0493	1	0.98438	0.01550	0.89422	0.99778
3	0.2849	1	0.96875	0.02175	0.88078	0.99209
4	0.4082	1	0.95313	0.02642	0.86168	0.98464
5	0.8767	1	0.93750	0.03026	0.84199	0.97607
6	0.8877	1	0.92188	0.03355	0.82244	0.96672
7	1.1233	1	0.90625	0.03644	0.80317	0.95675
8	1.2247	0	0.90625	0.03675	0.80194	0.95705
9	1.3753	1	0.89035	0.03940	0.78265	0.94645
10	1.5425	1	0.87445	0.04178	0.76367	0.93542
11	1.5836	1	0.85855	0.04394	0.74497	0.92404
12	1.7397	1	0.84265	0.04591	0.72654	0.91234
13	1.7589	1	0.82675	0.04772	0.70836	0.90035
14	1.7726	1	0.81086	0.04938	0.69040	0.88811
15	1.9233	1	0.79496	0.05091	0.67265	0.87565
16	1.9562	0	0.79496	0.05142	0.67117	0.87629
17	2.0493	1	0.77873	0.05287	0.65326	0.86339
18	2.2986	1	0.76251	0.05420	0.63555	0.85028
19	2.3425	1	0.74629	0.05542	0.61802	0.83697
20	3.7315	1	0.73006	0.05654	0.60066	0.82349
21	4.0548	1	0.71384	0.05757	0.58347	0.80984
22	4.0685	0	0.71384	0.05823	0.58177	0.81076
23	4.5863	1	0.69724	0.05920	0.56435	0.79666
24	4.9534	1	0.68064	0.06007	0.54709	0.78239
25	5.1534	0	0.68064	0.06082	0.54524	0.78346
26	5.7315	0	0.68064	0.06159	0.54332	0.78456
27	5.8493	1	0.66318	0.06244	0.52537	0.76946
28	5.8685	1	0.64573	0.06319	0.50759	0.75419
29	6.0712	0	0.64573	0.06406	0.50550	0.75548
30	6.1151	0	0.64573	0.06497	0.50333	0.75681
31	7.3781	0	0.64573	0.06591	0.50105	0.75819
32	7.6630	0	0.64573	0.06691	0.49867	0.75963
33	8.0438	0	0.64573	0.06794	0.49616	0.76113
34	8.1890	0	0.64573	0.06903	0.49354	0.76270
35	8.2055	0	0.64573	0.07017	0.49078	0.76433
36	8.2548	0	0.64573	0.07137	0.48786	0.76603
37	8.4274	0	0.64573	0.07263	0.48479	0.76782
38	8.4521	0	0.64573	0.07397	0.48154	0.76969
39	8.7589	0	0.64573	0.07538	0.47809	0.77165
40	9.0356	0	0.64573	0.07687	0.47443	0.77371
41	9.8959	0	0.64573	0.07845	0.47054	0.77589
42	9.9151	0	0.64573	0.08014	0.46638	0.77818
43	9.9178	0	0.64573	0.08194	0.46192	0.78061
44	10.1151	0	0.64573	0.08387	0.45714	0.78319
45	10.4027	0	0.64573	0.08594	0.45199	0.78592

46	10.6000	0	0.64573	0.08817	0.44642	0.78884
47	10.6603	1	0.61175	0.08984	0.41363	0.76065
48	10.6685	0	0.61175	0.09245	0.40743	0.76416
49	10.7260	0	0.61175	0.09529	0.40063	0.76795
50	10.9260	0	0.61175	0.09842	0.39316	0.77205
51	10.9370	0	0.61175	0.10187	0.38489	0.77651
52	11.2027	0	0.61175	0.10572	0.37567	0.78139
53	11.4548	0	0.61175	0.11004	0.36532	0.78676
54	11.4712	0	0.61175	0.11493	0.35359	0.79270
55	11.5589	0	0.61175	0.12054	0.34016	0.79934
56	11.6082	0	0.61175	0.12706	0.32460	0.80683
57	11.6164	0	0.61175	0.13477	0.30631	0.81536
58	11.6521	0	0.61175	0.14407	0.28446	0.82522
59	11.7123	0	0.61175	0.15562	0.25784	0.83679
60	11.7671	0	0.61175	0.17047	0.22465	0.85066
61	11.8466	0	0.61175	0.19059	0.18222	0.86775
62	11.8575	0	0.61175	0.22007	0.12703	0.88954
63	11.8685	0	0.61175	0.26953	0.05793	0.91871
64	11.9863	0	0.61175	0.38118	0.00274	0.95988
65	12.0082	0	0.61175	.	.	.

The macro KMPLOT is designed to be invoked immediately after KMTABLE. It allows the user to produce high-resolution graphs of the survival curves. Of course, it can be used only if SAS/GRAPH software is licensed. The following options can be used:

1. The confidence intervals calculated by KMTABLE may be plotted on the same graph as the survival curve.

2. The censored or complete times can be marked.

3. Multiple plots for distinct values of a BY variable specified in KMPLOT can be printed either separately or on the same graph. In the latter case, confidence intervals cannot also be produced because having multiple curves and their confidence intervals on the same graph would be confusing.

4. A cutoff condition such as $t < timeval$ or $r > n$ at risk can be specified to omit the extreme right hand tails from the curve(s) plotted.

A listing of KMPLOT is given at the end of this chapter.

The template given below makes it easier to use this macro.

```
%macro kmplot(
mark=                /* yes to mark times on curve,
                        no (default) to not mark times */
,ci=                 /* yes for confidence intervals,
                        no (default) for no ci's */
,combine=            /* yes to produce multiple plots
                        on the same graph, no (default)
                        for separate plots */
,xlabel=             /* label for the horizontal axis,
                        default is time */
,ylabel=             /* label for the vertical axis,
                        default is Pct Survival */
,title=              /* default is Kaplan-Meier Survival Curve */
,cutoff=             /* clause to restrict curve(s), usually of form
                        time < value or r < value (for n at risk)*/
)
```

Example 2.3 shows how the macro KMPLOT can be invoked. It is assumed that you have previously invoked KMTABLE. Figure 2.4 is produced.

Example 2.3

```
%kmplot(
        mark= yes        /* yes to mark times on curve,
                            no (default) to not mark times */
        ,ci= yes         /* yes for confidence intervals,
                            no (default) for no ci's */
                         /* yes to produce multiple plots
                            on the same graph, no (default)
                            for separate plots */
                         /* label for the horizontal axis,
                            default is time */
                         /* label for the vertical axis,
                            default is Pct Survival */

        ,title= Figure 2.4 /* default is Kaplan-Meier Survival
                            Curve */
                             /* clause to restrict curve(s),
                                usually of form time < value or r
                            < value (for n at risk)*/
```

or equivalently

```
%kmplot(mark=yes, ci=yes, title=Figure 2.4)
```

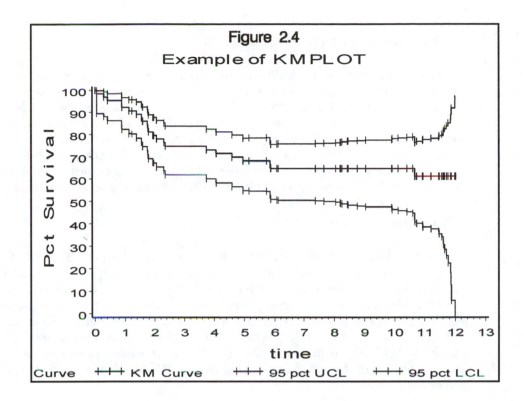

Figure 2.4
Example of KM PLOT

9. Planning a Study to Control the Standard Error

9.1 General Considerations

When estimating parameters from sample data, we would generally present not only those estimates, but also some additional information that provides some idea as to their precision. This is usually done by reporting the standard error of the estimates or confidence intervals for the parameters being studied. If you are working with data that have previously been collected, you have no control of that precision. On the other hand, when asked to plan a study whose purpose is estimation, you can recommend study characteristics that can be expected to provide a desired level of precision for the estimates obtained. In many situations, the only relevant study characteristic is the sample size. For example, biostatisiticians are constantly asked to calculate the sample size needed to produce an estimator of a mean or proportion that will have sufficiently small standard error.

9.2 The Survival Analysis Situation

When estimating survival probabilities, however, the situation is a bit more complicated. The standard error of such estimates will, in general, depend not only on the sample size, but also on the rate and pattern of the patients' entry onto the study and the distribution of losses to follow-up. This section shows how to predict, based on these characteristics, the (Peto) standard error of Kaplan-Meier estimates of the survival distribution and presents a macro to perform the necessary calculations. While these calculations can be done for either the Greenwood or Peto variance formulas, they are much easier to do for the Peto formula. Thus, the discussion is based on that variance estimation formula.

9.3 Derivation of the Formula

The estimated variance of $\hat{S}(t)$, as given by Peto's formula, is $[\hat{S}(t)]^2[1 - \hat{S}(t)]/R(t)$ where $R(t)$ is the number at risk at time t. Thus, predicting that variance in advance, based on specific study characteristics, requires some prediction of $\hat{S}(t)$, the proportion surviving at least to time t, and $R(t)$, the number whose time on study is at least t. The prediction of $\hat{S}(t)$ is not as critical as it may appear, so it will be discussed later. Focus for now on $R(t)$. Let N be the sample size and $P_R(t)$ be the probability that a subject is at risk, that is, alive and on study t units of time after entry. Then, a reasonable prediction for $R(t)$ is N times $P_R(t)$. Now, a person is at risk for time t if and only if all of the following three conditions are true:

1.   The subject's survival time is at least t.

2.   The subject entered the study early enough to be followed for time t.

3.   The subject was not lost or otherwise removed from the study prior to time t.

Because these can be thought of as independent events, their joint probability is the product of their individual probabilities. The first of these is estimated by $\hat{S}(t)$. The second depends on the pattern of the patients' entry onto the study and the additional follow-up time after patients are no longer being entered. Often patients enter for a set amount of time, T, and these entries are assumed to take place uniformly in $(0, T)$. Follow-up continues for an additional period of time, τ. If t is less than or equal to τ, then the probability of entering early enough to be at risk for time t is 1. Otherwise, a subject, to be at risk for time t, would have had to enter prior to time $T + \tau - t$. Assuming uniform patient entry, that probability is $(T + \tau - t)/T$. For the third probability, assume that the time until a patient is lost to follow-up is exponential with some constant rate, θ. Thus, the probability of not being lost to follow-up for time t is $\exp(-\theta t)$. Putting all of this together, we have

$$P_R(t) = \frac{\hat{S}(t)(T + \tau - t)\exp(-\theta t)}{T} \quad \text{if } t > \tau \tag{7}$$

$$= \exp(-\theta t) \quad \text{otherwise}$$

Thus, the standard error of $\hat{S}(t)$ is given (approximately) by

$$\sqrt{\frac{T\hat{S}(t)[1 - \hat{S}(t)]}{N(T + \tau - t)\exp(-\theta t)}} \quad \text{if } t > \tau$$

$$(8)$$

$$\sqrt{\frac{\hat{S}(t)[1 - \hat{S}(t)]}{N\exp(-\theta t)}} \quad \text{otherwise}$$

9.4 Dealing with $\hat{S}(t)$

Now consider the factor $\hat{S}(t)[1 - \hat{S}(t)]$. It's not difficult to see that it takes on its largest possible value of 0.25 when $\hat{S}(t)$ is 0.5. Also, it is larger for values of $\hat{S}(t)$ closer to 0.5. This enables us to replace $\hat{S}(t)$ in the above formula by a value that provides a conservative estimate. The potential error in using 0.5 for $\hat{S}(t)$ is not too bad if $\hat{S}(t)$ turns out to be reasonably close to that value. For $\hat{S}(t) = 0.5, \sqrt{\hat{S}(t)[1 - \hat{S}(t)]} = 0.5$. For $\hat{S}(t) = 0.7$, it is about 0.46.

9.5 An Example

Suppose that one of the primary objectives of a study you are planning is to estimate survival probabilities over time for patients with advanced Hodgkin's disease who are receiving an experimental treatment regimen. You expect to be able to accrue 30 patients per year, that a five-year survival will be between 60% and 80%, and that about 5% will drop out or be lost to follow-up in a year. This last assumption allows us to use $\theta = 0.05$. (More precisely, you could use $\theta = -\log_e(0.95) = 0.0513$, but such precision is not needed.) You would like to predict the standard error of $\hat{S}(5)$ if you accrue for four years and follow patients for three years more before performing the analysis. Taking $\hat{S}(5) = 0.6$, $N = 120$, $T = 4$, $\tau = 3$, $t = 5$, and $\theta = 0.05$, you obtain a predicted standard deviation of about 0.056. If this value is larger than you would like, you must consider increasing the accrual rate, the accrual time, or the follow-up time.

9.6 The KMPLAN Macro

The macro KMPLAN calculates the (Peto) predicted standard error of $\hat{S}(t)$ for a given value of t and values of the accrual rate, the accrual time, the follow-up time, $S(t)$, and the loss rate, θ. The parameters ACCTIME, FUTIME, and ACCRATE can be specified as specific values or ranges (for example, ACCTIME=3 to 5 or ACCRATE=50 TO 100 BY 50). Note that if losses to follow-up are not anticipated, then $\theta = 0$ can be used. In fact, this is the default value for this parameter. The default value of $S(t)$ is 0.5. A listing of this macro appears at the end of this chapter.

To use this macro, you can fill in the parameters in the template below:

```
%kmplan(
        acctime=              /*accrual time, can be range*/
        ,futime=              /*post-accrual follow-up
                                time, can be range*/
        ,accrate=             /*accrual rate, can be range*/
        ,lossrate=            /*loss rate, default is 0*/

        ,t=                   /*t for which projected se of
                                KM estimate of S(t) is wanted*/
        ,s=                   /*assumed value of S(t), default
                                0.5 which is conservative*/
    )
```

9.7 An Example of the Use of KMPLAN

Suppose you are planning a study whose major objective is to estimate survival probabilities over time for patients with a life threatening condition who are given an experimental treatment. You would like to assure that $S(3)$, the three-year survival rate, is estimated with a standard error not exceeding 3%. You believe that your institution can accrue 20 patients per year, but it is possible to add one or two additional institutions that can also accrue 20 patients per year. $S(3)$ is expected to be between 40% and 60%, so you can use the default value of 50%. A loss rate of 5% per year can be expected. Example 2.4 shows how to use KMPLAN to produce estimates of the projected standard error over a range of possible choices for the study parameters.

Example 2.4

```
%kmplan(
        acctime=4 to 6    /*accrual time, can be range*/
        ,futime=2 to 4    /*post-accrual follow-up
                            time, can be range*/
        ,accrate=20 to 60 by 20 /*accrual rate, can be range*/
        ,lossrate=.05     /*loss rate, default is 0*/

        ,t=3              /*t for which projected se of
                            KM estimate of S(t) is wanted*/
                          /*assumed value of S(t), default
                            0.5 which is conservative*/
        )
```

or equivalently

```
%kmplan(acctime=4 to 6, futime=2 to 4, accrate=20 to 60 by 20,
        lossrate=.05, t=3)
```

Using KMPLAN as indicated above produces Output 2.3.

Output 2.3

```
              Projected Standard Error (Peto) of Kaplan-Meier
                    Estimate of Survival at t = 3 Assuming
                       S(3) = .5 and Loss Rate of 0.05


                                                        Projected
         Accrual       Accrual     Follow-up    Sample   Standard
          Rate          Time         Time        Size     Error


           20            4            2           80     0.049198
           20            4            3           80     0.042607
           20            4            4           80     0.042607
           20            5            2          100     0.042607
           20            5            3          100     0.038109
           20            5            4          100     0.038109
           20            6            2          120     0.038109
           20            6            3          120     0.034789
           20            6            4          120     0.034789
           40            4            2          160     0.034789
           40            4            3          160     0.030128
           40            4            4          160     0.030128
           40            5            2          200     0.030128
           40            5            3          200     0.026947
           40            5            4          200     0.026947
           40            6            2          240     0.026947
           40            6            3          240     0.024599
           40            6            4          240     0.024599
           60            4            2          240     0.028405
           60            4            3          240     0.024599
           60            4            4          240     0.024599
           60            5            2          300     0.024599
           60            5            3          300     0.022002
           60            5            4          300     0.022002
           60            6            2          360     0.022002
           60            6            3          360     0.020085
           60            6            4          360     0.020085
```

You can see from the results above that, even with six years of accrual and four additional years of follow-up, you do not achieve the desired standard error with only one institution and an accrual rate of 20 per year. With two institutions, it appears that four years of accrual and three additional years of follow-up will suffice.

9.8 Some Observations about the Results

It is interesting to note that an additional year of follow-up apparently does not produce a smaller estimated standard error for $\hat{S}(3)$. This might lead one to conclude that the additional year of follow-up would not contribute to the study. That would not be correct. Recall that the conservatism of Peto's formula for the standard error of $\hat{S}(t)$ is due to the fact that it is based only on the number of patients at risk for time t. In fact, patients who are observed for less time are counted in calculating $\hat{S}(t)$ as well, and they contribute to its precision. Also, keep in mind that, although the study is being planned so that the standard error of the three-year estimate is controlled, you will also be reporting estimates for longer periods of time. Longer follow-up will improve the precision of those estimates as well.

Another apparently incongruous result is that with an accrual rate of 40 patients per year, you seem to have the same standard error for five years of accrual and two years of follow-up as for four years of accrual and three years of follow-up. It appears that the additional 20 patients accrued in the first plan do not contribute to the study. Again, this is due to the conservatism of the formula used. Of the 200 patients accrued in five years with two years of follow-up, only the 160 accrued during the first four years could be at risk for three years. All of the 160 accrued in four years with three years of follow-up could be at risk for three years. Of course, with five years of accrual, you would have 40 additional patients at risk for less time than that. Their contribution to the precision of $\hat{S}(3)$ is not reflected in Peto's formula.

10. Interval Censored Data

10.1 Interval Censoring

Sometimes, when dealing with survival data, patients are assessed for the endpoint under study only sporadically. Thus, you may only know that the i'th patient achieved the endpoint at a time in the interval $(L_i, R_i]$. Here L_i can be 0 and R_i can be infinite. If these intervals are not too wide, most analysts would simply treat such an observation as if it occurred at time R_i. For example, if a cancer patient was free of disease at time 3.4 and is found to have relapsed when evaluated at time 3.9, that patient would have an event time of 3.9. A consequence of this is that reported survival results can be influenced by the frequency with which patients are evaluated for the endpoint being studied.

10.2 The ICE Macro

Peto (1973) and Turnbull (1976) discuss a method of dealing with interval censored data such as that described above. The method is quite complicated and produces estimates that may not be defined in certain intervals. A macro, named ICE, which performs the required computations can be found in the SAS/IML sample library in Release 6.11 or later. Finding it may be a little tricky. If you are using the Windows version of SAS software, Release 6.11 or later, you get to the sample library by clicking on Help. Then choose Sample Programs, SAS Sample Library, and SAS/IML. Finally, click on Interval Censored Estimation Macro. You will then see the ICE macro on the screen. Save it by using copy/paste. The ICE macro uses some utilities that are contained in the XMACRO.SAS file, so you will need it as well. The file, XMACRO.SAS is found in the sample subdirectory. Other versions of SAS software have a subdirectory of sample programs in the IML subdirectory. The ICE macro can be found there. Again, you will need to find the XMACRO.SAS file as well. If you can't find these files or if you are using Release version 6.08 to 6.10, you can download both files from the World Wide Web. Use the search tool on the SAS Institute homepage at http://www.sas.com. The program does not work with SAS releases prior to 6.08.

10.3 Using the ICE Macro

In order to use the ICE macro, your data must contain two time variables. For (right, left, or interval) censored data, these two variables give the left and right endpoints of the interval in which the event is known to have occurred. If these variable names are, for example, L and R then L can be zero for a left censored observation. For a right censored observation, you can take R to be some arbitrary large number that is larger than the largest observed time. If an event time is known, you take L and R both equal to that time. The macro permits the use of several optional arguments. Many are rather technical and allow you to control the method and details of the likelihood maximization. The defaults will usually work fine, so these arguments won't be discussed here. The following arguments may be useful:

DATA= The name of the SAS data set to be used. The default is to use the last data set defined.

BY= An optional list of BY variables. If this is used, then the ice macro produces separate analyses for each combination of by variable values.

TIME= This is the only argument that is required. It gives the names of the variables representing the left and right endpoints of the time interval. They may be enclosed in parentheses, brackets, or braces, but that is not necessary.

FREQ= A numeric variable indicating the number of observations represented by an observation.

OPTIONS= This is a list of display options that you may use. If you use PLOT, you will get a graph of the survival curve.

Here are a couple of suggestions. The file MACRO.SAS contains a statement of the form

```
%include filename
```

where *filename* is the path and name of the file XMACRO.SAS. You may need to change this statement to conform to the path of XMACRO.SAS on your computer. Also, the ICE.SAS program contains the statement

```
call gdrawl(xy1,xy2)color="cyan";
```

This produces a graph with light blue lines that look fine on a color monitor or when printed by a color printer. With a black and white printer, however, they are difficult to see. If you intend to print the graph on such a printer, you might want to change the statement to

```
call gdrawl(xy1,xy2);
```

The default color will be black.

10.4 Example

Example 2.5 is the one given in the documentation provided with ICE.SAS. The only change I made was to use the OPTIONS=PLOT argument to get the graph of the survival function.

Example 2.5

```
data ex1;
        input l r f;
        cards;
0 2  1
1 3  1
2 10 4
4 10 4
;
run;
%ice(data=ex1, time=(l r), freq=f, options=plot)
```

The above data indicate that one patient died in less than two units of time and one died between times one and three. Four patients lived past time=2 and four lived part time=4. We cannot tell whether their times are right censored (i.e., known only to be greater than 10) or interval censored (i.e., between 2 and 10 or 4 and 10). The results are given in Output 2.4 and Figure 2.5.

Output 2.4

```
                        The SAS System

            Nonparametric Survival Curve for Interval Censoring




Number of Observations: 4
Number of Parameters: 3
Optimization Technique: Newton Raphson Ridge




                              Parameter Estimates
                          Q         P        THETA
                          1         2        0.1999995

                          2         3        0.0000010

                          4        10        0.7999995




        Survival Curve Estimates and 95% Confidence Intervals

     LEFT        RIGHT       ESTIMATE        LOWER          UPPER
       0           1         1.0000            .              .
       2           2         0.8000          0.4494         1.0000
       3           4         0.8000          0.4494         1.0000
      10          10         0.0000            .              .
```

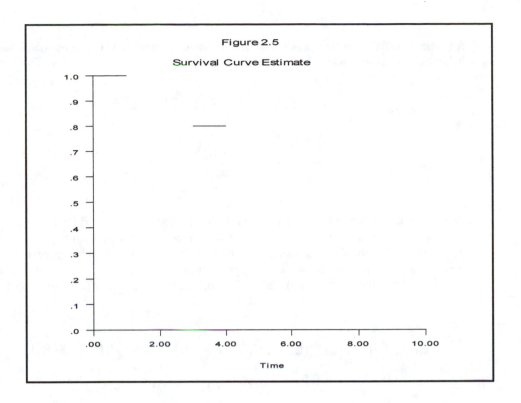

Figure 2.5

Survival Curve Estimate

10.5 Discussion of the Results

The results above give the estimated survival function as 1.0 for t between 0 and 1, as 0.8 for $t=2$ and for t between 3 and 4, and as 0.0 for $t = 10$. Note that survival estimates are not defined for t between 1 and 2 or t between 2 and 3. This illustrates the fact that the method of Peto and Turnbull may result in an estimated survival function that excludes certain intervals.

11.   Additional Details

11.1 The Delta Method

The delta method provides a way to estimate the variance of a random variable of the form $g(X)$ where X is a random variable whose variance is known and g is differentiable. For example, it is known that if X is the number of heads produced when ten unbiased coins are tossed, then the mean of X is five and its variance is 2.5. Now suppose you need to estimate the variance of $\exp(X)$. That's the sort of problem you can use the delta method for. This method is based on the Taylor formula for approximating an infinitely differentiable function by a polynomial.

It is shown in calculus that, under modest conditions, a function $g(x)$ can be written as an infinite series as follows:

$$g(x) = g(a) + \frac{g'(a)(x - a)}{1!} + \frac{g''(a)(x - a)^2}{2!} + \ldots$$

$$+ \frac{g^{(n)}(a)(x - a)^n}{n!} + \ldots$$

(9)

Where a is any real number. This is called the Taylor expansion of $g(x)$ about a. Truncating formula 9 at a finite number of terms gives an approximation of $g(x)$ by a polynomial. In particular, truncating after the first-degree term yields the approximation $g(x) \cong g(a) + g'(a)(x - a)$. Now if θ is any population parameter and $\hat{\theta}$ is an estimator of θ, this can be written $g(\hat{\theta}) \cong g(\theta) + g'(\theta)(\hat{\theta} - \theta)$. Taking variances of both sides, we have

$$var[g(\hat{\theta})] \approx var[g(\theta) + g'(\theta)(\hat{\theta} - \theta)] = var[g'(\theta)(\hat{\theta} - \theta)]$$

$$= [g'(\theta)]^2 var(\hat{\theta} - \theta)$$

(10)

Finally, noting that $var(\hat{\theta} - \theta) = var(\hat{\theta})$ and that $g'(\theta)$ can be approximated by $g'(\hat{\theta})$ we have the basic result

$$var[g(\hat{\theta})] \approx [g'(\hat{\theta})]^2 var(\hat{\theta})$$

(11)

This result is used twice below in the development of the formula for the variance of $\hat{S}(t)$. It is used several other times in this and later chapters.

11.2. Greenwood's Formula for the Variance of $\hat{S}(t)$

The estimate of the variance of $\hat{S}(t)$ to be presented below was originally described by Greenwood (1926) for the actuarial estimate of the survival function. It can be shown, however, that it is appropriate for the Kaplan-Meier estimate as well. Given below is a rough derivation of it, which treats certain quantities that are actually random as being constant and ignores the dependence of the factors in formula 1. A more complete argument is given by Miller (1981).

Begin by considering the variance of $\log_e \hat{S}(t)$. Taking the natural logarithm of both sides of formula 1, we obtain

$$\log_e[\hat{S}(t)] = \sum_{t_i \leq t} \log_e \frac{r_i - d_i}{r_i} \tag{12}$$

Now each $(r_i - d_i)/r_i$ can be thought of as an estimate of a proportion. Hence, its variance is estimated by $[(r_i - d_i)d_i]/r_i^3$. Using the delta method, the variance of $\log_e[(r_i - d_i)d_i]/r_i^3$ can be estimated by $\{(r_i - d_i)/r_i\}^{-2}\{[(r_i - d_i)d_i]/r_i^3\}$. Thus we have

$$var[\log_e \hat{S}(t)] \approx \sum_{t_i \leq t} \frac{d_i}{r_i(r_i - d_i)} \tag{13}$$

Again, we apply the delta method, this time to estimate $var[\hat{S}(t)]$ as $var\{\exp[\log_e \hat{S}(t)]\}$. The final result is

$$var[\hat{S}(t)] \approx [\hat{S}(t)]^2 \sum_{t_i \leq t} \frac{d_i}{r_i(r_i - 1)} \tag{14}$$

Formula 14 is known as Greenwood's formula for estimating the variance of $\hat{S}(t)$.

11.3 A Confidence Interval for S(t)

Let $V(t) = \log_e\{-\log_e[S(t)]\}$ and $\hat{V}(t) = \log_e\{-\log_e[\hat{S}(t)]\}$. Then, using the delta method, we have

$$var[\hat{V}(t)] \approx \frac{var[\hat{S}(t)]}{[\hat{S}(t)\log_e \hat{S}(t)]^2} \tag{15}$$

Denote $var[\hat{V}(t)]$ by $s^2(t)$. Then $\hat{V}(t) \pm z_{\alpha/2}s(t)$ is an approximate $(1-\alpha)100\%$ confidence interval for $V(t)$. Applying the exponential function twice produces $\hat{S}(t)^{\exp(\pm x)}$ as an approximate $(1-\alpha)100\%$ confidence interval for $S(t)$ where $x = z_{\alpha/2}s(t)$.

11.4 The KMTABLE Macro

```
%macro kmtable(dataset=_last_          /* dataset used by macro */
               ,pct=95                 /* for conf. int. */
               ,time=                  /* time variable */
               ,cens=                  /* variable that indicates
                                          censored or complete time */
               ,censval=               /* value(s) that indicate
                                          censored time */
               ,method=                /* 1 for conf. int. method used
                                          in Proc Lifetest, 2 for
                                          method that yields limits in
                                          (0,1) */
               ,variance=              /* G or g for Greenwood=s
                                          formula, P or p for Peto=s
                                          formula */
               ,byvar=none             /* Optional by variable(s) for
                                          separate tables */
               ,print=yes              /* no to suppress printing */
);
%global byvari perc ttime;
%let byvari=&byvar;
%let perc=&pct;
%let ttime=&time;
data &dataset;
        set &dataset;
        none=1;
run;
proc sort data=&dataset;
        by &byvar;
run;

/*  Create dataset, x, with survival estimates */
proc lifetest noprint outs=x data=&dataset;
        by &byvar;
        time &time*&cens(&censval);
run;
proc sort out=y;
        by &byvar &time;
run;
/* Add number at risk, r, to dataset */
data y;
        set y;
        by &byvar;
        if first.&byvar then r=0;
        else r+1;
        keep r &byvar;
run;
/* Merge number at risk with survival estimates */
proc sort;
        by &byvar descending r;
run;
data table;
        merge x y;
run;
proc sort;
        by &byvar descending r;
run;
/* Create Life Table */
data table;
        set table;
        by &byvar;
            /* Allow for G or P, check for valid values,
               if mis-specified, set values and put
               warning in log.                         */
        if _n_ = 1 then do;
        %if &variance = G %then %let variance=g;
        %if &variance = P %then %let variance=p;
        if "&variance" not in ('g', 'p') then do;
                put;
                put '***********************************';
                put '*Note: Invalid value of variance used*';
                put '*for choice of variance formula.  g *';
                put '*for Greenwood will be used.        *';
                put '***********************************';
                put;
        end;
end;
```

```
           if &method not in (1, 2) then do;
                 put;
                 put '**************************************';
                 put '*Note:  Invalid value of method used*';
                 put '*for choice of CI. Method 1 (as in  *';
                 put '*Proc Lifetest) will be used.       *';
                 put '**************************************';
                 put;
           end;
         end;
                  /* defaults for variance and conf int method */
         %if &variance ne g and &variance ne p %then
                 %let variance =g;
         %if &method ne 1 and &method ne 2 %then
                 %let method = 1;
                  /* normal critical value for conf. int. */
         z=-probit((100-&pct)/200);
         d=1-_censor_;
                  /* Peto s.e. */
         sp=survival*sqrt((1-survival)/r);
                  /* Greenwood s.e. */
         if first.&byvar then do;
          sum=0;
          stderr=0;
         end;
         else do;
          sum+d/(r*(r+1));
          sg=survival*sqrt(sum);
         end;
         if "&variance"='g'
                 then stderr=sg;
         if "&variance"='p'
                 then stderr=sp;
   /*  Confidence interval limits */
         if &method=1 then do;
          lcl=survival-z*stderr;
          lcl=max(0,lcl);
          ucl=survival+z*stderr;
          ucl=min(1.00, ucl);
         end;
         if &method=2 then do;
          s=-stderr/log(survival)/survival;
          lcl=survival**(exp(z*s));
          ucl=survival**(exp(-z*s));
         end;
         if first.&byvar then do;
          stderr=0;
          lcl=1;
          ucl=1;
         end;
   /*  Create column label for table */
         %if &variance=g %then
                 label stderr = 'Greenwood*stderr';;
         %if &variance = p %then
                 label stderr = 'Peto*stderr';;
         %if &method = 1 %then %do;
          label lcl= "Method 1*&pct pct lcl";;
          label ucl="Method 1*&pct pct ucl";;
         %end;
         %if &method =2 %then %do;
          label lcl = "Method 2*&pct pct lcl";;
          label ucl = "Method 2*&pct pct ucl";;
         %end;
run;
proc sort;
  by &byvar;
run;
/* Print life table  */
%if &print = yes %then %do;
         proc print l split='*';
         var  &time d survival stderr lcl ucl;
   %if &byvar ne none %then by &byvar;;
%end;
run;
%mend kmtable;
```

11.5 The KMPLOT Macro

```
%macro kmplot(mark=no                          /*  yes to mark times
                                                    on curve */
              ,ci=no                           /*  yes for conf.
                                                    intervals */
              ,ylabel= Pct Survival            /*  label for y axis */
              ,xlabel=time                     /*  label for x axis */
              ,combine=no                      /*  yes to put multiple
                                                    plots on same
                                                    graph */
              ,cutoff=none                     /*  clause to restrict
                                                    curve(s), usually
                                                    of form time<value
                                                    or r<value (for n
                                                    at risk) */
              ,title= Kaplan-Meier Survival Curve
);
/* no conf. interval if multiple plots on graph */
%if &combine=yes %then %let ci=no;;
/* Define symbol statements */
%if &combine&mark=yesno %then %do;
   symbol1 l=1 f= , v=none  i=stepjl w=5;
        symbol2 l=3 f= ,v=none i=stepjl w=5;
        symbol3 l=5 f= ,v=none i=stepjl w=5;
        symbol4 l=33 f= ,v=none i=stepjl w=5;
             %end;
%if &combine&mark=yesyes %then %do;
        symbol1 l=1 f=swiss v="|" i=stepjl w=5;
        symbol2 l=3 f=swiss v="|" i=stepjl w=5;
        symbol3 l=5 f=swiss v="|" i=stepjl w=5;
        symbol4 l=33 f=swiss v="|" i=stepjl w=5;
  %end;

%if &combine&mark=noyes %then %do;
        symbol1 l=1 f=swiss v="|" i=stepjl w=5;
        symbol2 l=3 f= ,v=none i=stepjl w=5;
        symbol3 l=3 f= ,v=none i=stepjl w=5;
%end;
%if &combine&mark=nono %then %do;
        symbol1 l=1 f= , v=none i=stepjl w=5;
        symbol2 l=3 f= , v=none i=stepjl w=5;
        symbol3 l=3 f= , v=none i=stepjl w=5;
   %end;
/* White out by if no by variables */
%if &byvari=none %then goptions cby=white;;
/* Create dataset for plot(s) */
data;
        set table;
        survival=survival*100;
        lcl=100*lcl;
        ucl=100*ucl;
        y=survival;
        curve=1;
        output;
        y=ucl;
        curve=2;
        %if &ci=yes %then output;;
        y=lcl;
        curve=3;
        %if &ci=yes %then output;;
run;
proc sort;
  by &byvari curve &ttime;
run;
proc format;
  value curve 1='KM curve' 2='UCL' 3='LCL';
run;
/* Define axes and legends */
axis1 width=5 minor=none
        label=(h=3 f=swissb a=90 j=center
        "&ylabel")
        value = ( h=1.5 f=swissb) order=(0 to 100 by 10);
axis2 width=5
        label=(h=3 f=swissb  "&xlabel")
        value=(h=1.5 f=swissb);
```

```
%if &combine=no %then
        legend1 label= (f=swissb h=1.5  'Curve')
        value=(f=swissb h=1.5 j=l 'KM Curve' "&perc pct UCL" "&perc
pct    LCL");;
legend2 label=(f=swissb h=1.5)
        value=(f=swissb h=1.5 j=l);
%if &combine=no %then %do;

/* gplot for separate curves */
        proc gplot;
            %if &cutoff ne none %then where &cutoff;;
        plot y*time= curve /
        legend=legend1
        vaxis=axis1 haxis=axis2
        %if &ci=no %then nolegend;;
        ;
        by &byvari;
        format curve curve.;
%end;
run;
 %if &combine=yes %then %do;
/* gplot for combined curves */
        proc gplot;
            %if &cutoff ne none %then where &cutoff;;
            plot y*time=&byvari/ legend=legend2
        vaxis=axis1 haxis=axis2;
        %end;
title &title;
run;
%mend kmplot;
```

11.6 The KMPLAN Macro

```
%macro kmplan(
            acctime=            /*  accrual time, can be range */
            ,futime=            /*  post-accrual follow-up time, can
                                    be range */
            ,accrate=           /*  accrual rate, can be range */
            ,lossrate=0         /*  loss rate */
            ,s=.5               /*  assumed value of S(t) */
            ,t=                 /*  time for which projected se is
                                    wanted */
) ;
data out;
/* define variables from arguments in macro */
        s = &s;
        t = &t;
        lossrate=&lossrate;
/* start loops for study parameters */
        do accrate = &accrate;
        do acctime = &acctime;
      do futime = &futime;
  /* calculate Peto standard error */
        x = 1;
        if t > futime then
            x = (acctime + futime - t)/acctime;
        n = accrate*acctime;
        stderr = s*sqrt((1 - s)/(n*x*exp(-lossrate*t)));
        output;
      end;
    end;
end;
run;
/* Create column labels */
label acctime = 'Accrual Time';
label futime = 'Follow-up Time';
label n = 'Sample Size';
label accrate = 'Accrual Rate';
label stderr = 'Projected Standard Error';
```

```
/* print with titles */
proc print noobs l;
        var accrate acctime futime n stderr;
        title 'Projected Standard Error (Peto) of Kaplan-Meier';
        title2 "Estimate of Survival at t = &t Assuming";
        title3 " S(&t) = &s and Loss Rate of &lossrate";
run;
%mend kmplan;
```

Chapter 3   Nonparametric Comparison of Survival Distributions

1. Notation

In this chapter you will learn how to compare two or more groups with respect to survival. Although it would be possible to jump right into the more general discussion of K groups for any integer $K > 1$, the exposition will be more clear if the initial presentation is for $K = 2$ groups. The generalization to $K > 2$ will then be straightforward.

First, some slight modifications to previous notation are needed. Label the groups being compared 1 and 2, and assume that they have unknown survival functions $S_1(t)$ and $S_2(t)$ respectively. Suppose you have samples of sizes N_1 and N_2 from these groups. Let $N = N_1 + N_2$ and let $t_1 < t_2 < \ldots < t_M$ be the distinct ordered censored or complete times for the combined sample. There may be ties so that $M \le N$. For each i from 1 to M and for $j = 1$ or 2, let d_{ij} be the number of deaths in group j at time t_i and let $d_i = d_{i1} + d_{i2}$. That is, d_{i1} is the number of deaths in group 1, d_{i2} is the number of deaths in group 2, and d_i is the total number of deaths in both groups at time t_i. Since we are allowing for ties, d_{i1}, d_{i2}, and d_i may be greater than 1. Let R_{ij} be the number at risk in group j just prior to time t_i and let $R_i = R_{i1} + R_{i2}$. As an example, suppose that in group 1 you have times 3, 5, 8+, 10, and 15, and in group 2 you have times 2, 5, 11+, 13+, 14, and 16, where times followed by a plus sign are censored. You can then represent these data in the following table:

Table 3.1

i	t_i	d_{i1}	d_{i2}	d_i	R_{i1}	R_{i2}	R_i
1	2	0	1	1	5	6	11
2	3	1	0	1	5	5	10
3	5	1	1	2	4	5	9
4	8	0	0	0	3	4	7
5	10	1	0	1	2	4	6
6	11	0	0	1	1	4	5
7	13	0	0	0	1	3	4
8	14	0	1	1	1	2	3
9	15	1	0	1	1	1	2
10	16	0	1	1	0	1	1

The shading in the previous table shows the group(s) for each observation time as indicated in the following legend:

Figure 3.1

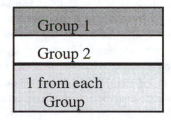

2. The Log Rank Statistic

2.1 Historical Background

The log rank statistic is a straightforward extension of concepts introduced by Mantel and Haenszel (1959). That paper shows how independent two by two contingency tables can be combined to generate one overall statistic. For this reason, the log rank statistic is often referred to as the Mantel-Haenszel statistic. The use of this idea to compare survival distributions was first presented by Mantel (1966). The term *log rank* comes from a paper by Peto and Peto (1972), in which they develop the statistic by considering an estimate of the logarithms of survival functions.

2.2 A Heuristic Development of the Statistic

At each time t_i, where i goes from 1 to M, we have d_i deaths, of which d_{i1} are from group 1 and d_{i2} are from group 2. These deaths occur among the R_i patients at risk at time t_i, of whom R_{i1} are in group 1 and R_{i2} are in group 2. If the two groups are equivalent with respect to survival, we would expect these deaths to be apportioned between those groups according to each group's proportion of the number at risk at that time. That is, the $E_{i1} = d_i R_{i1} / R_i$ expected values of d_{i1} and d_{i2} are $d_i R_{i1}/R_i$ and $d_i R_{i2}/R_i$, respectively under the null hypothesis that $S_1(t)$ is equivalent to $S_2(t)$ conditioned on the fact their total is d_i. We will denote these quantities by E_{i1} and E_{i2}. Then $d_{i1} - E_{i1}$ is a measure of how well or poorly group 1 did at time t_i compared with group 2. If $d_{i1} - E_{i1} > 0$, then group 1 experienced more deaths than expected at this time and if $d_{i1} - E_{i1} < 0$, then group 1 experienced fewer deaths than expected at this time. Similar statements can be made about $d_{i2} - E_{i2}$. Now let $d_{.1} = \Sigma d_{i1}$, $d_{.2} = \Sigma d_{i2}$, $E_1 = \Sigma E_{i1}$, and $E_2 = \Sigma E_{i2}$, where all of these sums are taken over $i = 1, 2, \ldots, M$. Then $d_{.1} - E_1$, which equals $\Sigma(d_{i1} - E_{i1})$, is a statistic that measures how well or poorly group 1 did compared with group 2 over the entire course of the study. The remaining problem, of course, is to be able to say something about the distribution of this statistic so that we can determine whether or not it offers strong evidence that one group has better survival than the other. This problem is discussed in the next section.

2.3. Two Alternatives

One way to evaluate the significance of the statistic $d_{.1} - E_1$ is to note that, following general principles for statistics of this kind, $(d_{.1} - E_1)^2/E_1 + (d_{.2} - E_2)^2/E_2$ has, *asymptotically* (that is, approximately for large samples), a χ^2 distribution with 1 degree of freedom under the null hypothesis of equivalent survival distributions. Since the numerators of this statistic must be equal, this can be written as $(d_{.1} - E_1)^2(1/E_1 + 1/E_2)$. Another approach is to note that each of the $d_{i1} - E_{i1}$ have (under the null hypothesis) zero means as does their sum, $d_{.1} - E_1$. The variances of each of the $d_{i1} - E_{i1}$ are equal to $v_i = [R_{i1}R_{i2}d_i(R_i - d_i)]/[R_i^2(R_i - 1)]$. This is a consequence of the fact that, conditional on d_i, d_{i1} has a hypergeometric distribution. Although the $d_{i1} - E_{i1}$ are not independent, it can be shown that the variance of $\Sigma(d_{i1} - E_{i1}) = d_{.1} - E_1$ is approximately equal to the sum of the v_i's. Furthermore, $d_{.1} - E_1$ has, for reasonably large sample sizes, a distribution that is approximately normal. Thus we can compare $(d_{.1} - E_1)/(\Sigma v_i)^{1/2}$ to a standard normal distribution. These two approaches to testing the equivalence of two survival distributions can, therefore, be described as follows:

1. Calculate $(d_{.1} - E_1)^2(1/E_1 + 1/E_2)$. Reject the null hypothesis of equivalent survival distributions at the α significance level if its value exceeds the $(1 - \alpha)100$th percentile of a χ^2 distribution with 1 degree of freedom. For $\alpha = 0.05$, that value is 3.84.

2. Calculate $(d_{.1} - E_1)/(\Sigma v_i)^{1/2}$. Reject the null hypothesis of equivalent survival distributions at the α significance level if its absolute value exceeds the $(1 - \alpha/2)100$th percentile of a standard normal distribution. For $\alpha = 0.05$, that value is 1.96.

Since the $(1 - \alpha)100$th percentile of a χ^2 distribution with 1 degree of freedom equals the square of the $(1 - \alpha/2)100$th percentile of a standard normal distribution, approach 2 is equivalent to comparing $(d_{.1} - E_1)^2/(\Sigma v_i)$ to the same critical value as the statistic in approach 1. Thus, it is clear these two approaches differ only in that $(d_{.1} - E_1)^2$ is divided by $(1/E_1 + 1/E_2)^{-1}$ in the first case, and Σv_i in the second. Since it can be shown that $(1/E_1 + 1/E_2)^{-1} \geq \Sigma v_i$, the first approach will produce a smaller statistic and hence a more conservative test. Both approaches can be found in the literature on the subject and the formula $(d_{.1} - E_1)^2(1/E_1 + 1/E_2)$ was used in the SURVTEST procedure, a predecessor of the LIFETEST procedure. PROC LIFETEST uses the formula $(d_{.1} - E_1)/(\Sigma v_i)^{1/2}$. That formula is used here and as a basis for generalizations that follow.

2.4 An Example Using the Log Rank Statistic

Table 3.2 illustrates the calculation of the log rank statistic for the small samples discussed earlier in this chapter. The reader is cautioned that, because the approximation of the distribution of both statistics described in the previous section are approximately valid only for reasonably large samples, it would not be appropriate to use them with such a small sample.

Table 3.2

i	t_i	d_{i1}	d_{i2}	d_i	R_{i1}	R_{i2}	R_i	E_{i1}	v_i
1	2	0	1	1	5	6	11	0.455	0.248
2	3	1	0	1	5	5	10	0.500	0.250
3	5	1	1	2	4	5	9	0.889	0.432
4	8	0	0	0	3	4	7	0.000	0.000
5	10	1	0	1	2	4	6	0.333	0.222
6	11	0	0	0	1	4	5	0.000	0.000
7	13	0	0	0	1	3	4	0.000	0.000
8	14	0	1	1	1	2	3	0.333	0.222
9	15	1	0	1	1	1	2	0.500	0.250
10	16	0	1	1	0	1	1	0.000	0.000
Totals		4	4	8				3.010	1.624

From Table 3.2, you can calculate that $d_{.1} - E_1 = 0.990$ and $\Sigma v_i = 1.624$. The log rank statistic has the value of $0.990/1.624^{1/2} = 0.777$. Referring to a table of the standard normal distribution, you find a p-value for a two-sided test to be 0.437. As an alternative, you could obtain the same p-value by referring the value of $0.990^2/1.624$ to a χ^2 distribution with 1 degree of freedom. The conservative formula, $(d_{.1} - E_1)^2(1/E_1 + 1/E_2)$, leads to a p-value of 0.522.

Such values of the test statistic do not provide evidence to reject the null hypothesis that these two samples come from populations with equivalent survival. Recall, however, what was said earlier about the inadequacy of these sample sizes.

Notice that values of i for which $d_i = 0$ do not really enter into the calculation. For those lines of the table, d_{i1}, E_{i1}, and v_i are all 0. Thus the sums in Table 3.2 are often taken over only the times at which there is at least 1 death.

3. More Than Two Groups

3.1 Some New Notation

To generalize the result of the previous section's example to more than two groups requires some new notation. Suppose you have K groups whose unknown survival distributions are $S_1(t)$, $S_2(t)$, . . ., $S_K(t)$. Let N_j be the sample size in group j and $N = \Sigma N_j$. Again, let $t_1 < t_2 < . . . < t_M$ be the distinct ordered times in the combined sample. Extending the notation for two groups, R_{ij} is the number at risk in group j and R_i is the total number at risk just prior to time t_i. Also, d_{ij} is the number of deaths among those in group j, d_i is the total number of deaths, and $E_{ij} = d_i R_{ij}/R_i$ is the expected number of deaths in group j at time t_i. Then denote by $\mathbf{d}_i$ the column vector $(d_{i1}, d_{i2}, . . . d_{iK})'$ and by $\mathbf{E}_i$ the column vector $(E_{i1}, E_{i2}, . . . E_{iK})'$. Let $\mathbf{d}$ and $\mathbf{E}$ be the sums of the $\mathbf{d}_i$ and $\mathbf{E}_i$, respectively, over i. The vector $\mathbf{d} - \mathbf{E}$ is the generalization for $K > 2$ of the $d_{.1} - E_1$ that was used above for $K = 2$.

3.2 The Generalized Log Rank Statistic

In order to give the generalized log rank statistic for any $K > 2$, the estimated covariance matrix of the vector $\mathbf{d} - \mathbf{E}$ is needed. You can start with the variances and covariances for each i. The variance of $d_{ij} - E_{ij}$ can be estimated by

$$var_{ij} = \frac{d_i(R_i R_{ij} - R_{ij}^2)(R_i - d_i)}{R_i^2(R_i - 1)} \tag{1}$$

The covariance of $d_{ij} - E_{ij}$ and $d_{il} - E_{il}$ can be estimated by

$$cov_{ijl} = \frac{-R_{ij}R_{il}d_i(R_i - d_i)}{R_i^2(R_i - 1)} \tag{2}$$

The required variances and covariances for each entry of the covariance matrix of $\mathbf{d} - \mathbf{E}$ can then be estimated be summing these expressions over i. Since the components of $\mathbf{d} - \mathbf{E}$ must sum to zero, its covariance matrix will be singular. Let $\mathbf{S}$ be $\mathbf{d} - \mathbf{E}$ with one component removed, and let $\mathbf{V}$ be the covariance matrix of $\mathbf{S}$. Then if the j'th component is the one missing from $\mathbf{S}$, then $\mathbf{V}$ is simply the covariance matrix of $\mathbf{d} - \mathbf{E}$ with the j'th row and j'th column removed. $\mathbf{S}'\mathbf{V}^{-1}\mathbf{S}$ has, under the null hypothesis that all of the groups have equivalent survival, an asymptotic χ^2 distribution with $K-1$ degrees of freedom. It can be shown that the value of this statistic is the same regardless of which component of $\mathbf{d} - \mathbf{E}$ is omitted from $\mathbf{S}$. Note that the omission of a component generalizes the two-sample case in which the test statistic was based only on the deviation from expectation and the variance of that deviation in the first group. As in the two-sample case, you can instead base the test on the fact that the statistic

$(d_1 - E_1)^2/E_1 + (d_2 - E_2)^2/E_2 + \ldots + (d_K - E_K)^2/E_K$ has, asymptotically, a χ^2 distribution with $K - 1$ degrees of freedom under the null hypothesis. The resultant test will be conservative, as in the two-sample case. It does not require matrix inversion, however.

4. Other Linear Rank Tests

4.1 Weighted Sums

The log rank, or Mantel-Haenszel, test described in the previous two sections is actually just one realization of a general class of tests. Suppose we have, for each time, t_i, a weight, w_i. Instead of the statistic $\mathbf{d} - \mathbf{E}$ (which is the sum, over i, of the differences $\mathbf{d}_i - \mathbf{E}_i$), you can consider the weighted sum, $\Sigma w_i(\mathbf{d}_i - \mathbf{E}_i)$. Each component of that weighted sum is still a measure of the extent to which that group has survival that differs from its expectation under the null hypothesis. However, the log rank test (all $w_i = 1$) assigns the same weight to every death time. Other choices for the w_i assign differing weights to different death times. For example, if the w_i increase as i increases, then later death times affect the statistic more than earlier ones do. To calculate the covariance matrix of this weighted sum, simply multiply each component of the covariance matrix in the previous section by w_i^2. Thus, you now have

$$var_{ij} = \frac{w_i^2 d_i(R_i R_{ij} - R_{ij}^2)(R_i - d_i)}{R_i^2(R_i - 1)} \tag{3}$$

and

$$cov_{ijl} = \frac{-w_i^2 R_{ij} R_{il} d_i(R_i - d_i)}{R_i^2(R_i - 1)} \tag{4}$$

As in section 3.2, summing over i gives the variances and covariances of $\Sigma w_i(\mathbf{d}_i - \mathbf{E}_i)$. Letting $\mathbf{S}_w$ be the vector obtained by deleting one component from $\Sigma w_i(\mathbf{d}_i - \mathbf{E}_i)$ and $\mathbf{V}_w$ the covariance matrix formed by omitting the corresponding row and column from the covariance matrix of $\Sigma w_i(\mathbf{d}_i - \mathbf{E}_i)$, once again you can obtain the statistic $\mathbf{S}_w'\mathbf{V}_w^{-1}\mathbf{S}_w$ which, under the null hypothesis, has an asymptotic χ^2 distribution with $K-1$ degrees of freedom. In addition to the log rank test, several other tests, derived from other ways of defining the w_i's, have been presented by various authors. Such tests are known as *linear rank tests*.

4.2 Some Choices for Weights

Defining $w_i = R_i$ for all i gives you the Gehan test (1965). This test was originally described for two groups by Gehan as a generalization of the Wilcoxon rank sum test. For this reason, it is often known as the generalized Wilcoxon (or simply Wilcoxon) test. Breslow (1970) extended this test to K groups and, thus, it is sometimes known as the Breslow test. Because the w_i's are decreasing, this test gives greater weight to earlier deaths than does the log rank test. Tarone and Ware (1977) discuss weights defined by $w_i = R_i^{1/2}$. Still another choice, suggested by Harrington and Fleming (1982), is to assign weights equal to $[\hat{S}(t_i)]^\rho$ where the Kaplan-Meier estimate is based on the combined sample and ρ is a fixed nonnegative constant. This is a generalization of a test discussed by Prentice (1978) in which $\rho = 1$. Gray and Tsiatis (1989) discuss the interesting case of $K = 2$ and when the main interest is in comparing the cure rates of groups 1 and 2, assuming that survival among the non-cures is the same for both groups. In this case, they show that the asymptotically optimal weights w_i are the reciprocals of the Kaplan-Meier estimates at t_i. To avoid zero values of this estimate, they use what is often called the *left-continuous* version of this Kaplan-Meier estimator. In this version, the "step" in the estimated survival curve is defined to take place immediately after each death time instead of at that time.

Of course, the preceding paragraph raises the important question of which test, (that is, which set of weights) to use. Although all are valid, you should not compute more than one statistic and choose the one that is "most significant." You may, however, specify that the test be done based upon the way you expect the survival distributions to differ from the null hypothesis. For two groups, if the ratio of the hazards is constant over time (called the *proportional hazards assumption*) and the censoring distributions are the same, then the log rank test will have maximal power in the class of all linear rank tests (Peto and Peto, 1972). Perhaps for this reason, this test is the most frequently used. You may recall from Chapter 2 that the LIFETEST procedure provides a plot of the censoring times for each group. This plot provides a visual check of the assumption that the censoring distributions are the same. Lee et al. (1975) and Tarone and Ware (1977) show that when the proportional hazards assumption does not hold, other tests may have greater power. In general, only the Gehan and log rank tests are available in statistical software packages such as the SAS System. If the proportional hazards assumption seems tenable, then the log rank test is probably the best choice. Otherwise, you can perform power calculations for the most likely type of alternative by using a variety of test statistics and then choosing the statistic that most efficiently provides the greatest power or the desired power. This technique is discussed later in this chapter.

4.3 Summary

In conclusion, if $t_1, t_2, \ldots, t_M$ are the distinct death times, in ascending order, for patients in K groups and $w_1, w_2, \ldots, w_M$ are a set of weights, then the linear rank test, determined by these weights, at significance level α is performed as follows:

1. Form a table like the one in section 3. There should be a line for each time, t_i, at which a death occurred. The i'th line should contain, for each group j, the number of deaths, d_{ij}, in group j at time t_i, and R_{ij}, the number still at risk in group j just prior to time t_i. This line should also contain, for each group j, $E_{ij} = d_i R_{ij}/R_i$ where d_i and R_i are the sums of the d_{ij} and R_{ij} in the i'th row, and var_{ij} as defined by equation 3.

2. Let $\mathbf{d}_i$ be the vector $(d_{i1}, d_{i2}, \ldots d_{iK})'$ and $\mathbf{E}_i$ be the vector $(E_{i1}, E_{i2}, \ldots E_{iK})'$. Form the vector sum, $\Sigma w_i(\mathbf{d}_i - \mathbf{E}_i)$ and the j sums (over i), Σvar_{ij}.

3. For each pair of distinct groups j and l, and each row i, calculate cov_{ijl} as in equation 4. For each pair j and l, form the sums (over i) Σcov_{ijl}.

4. Form the K by K matrix in which the j'th main diagonal element is given by the the j'th sum, Σvar_{ij} and the j,l off-diagonal entry is given by the sum Σcov_{ijl}.

5. Form the vector $\mathbf{S}_w$ by removing one component from the vector $\Sigma w_i(\mathbf{d}_i - \mathbf{E}_i)$. Form the $(K-1)$ by $(K-1)$ matrix $\mathbf{V}_w$ by removing from the matrix formed in step 4, the row and column correspond to that same component.

6. Calculate $\mathbf{S}_w' \mathbf{V}_w^{-1} \mathbf{S}_w$ and compare it to the $(1-\alpha)100$th percentile of a χ^2 distribution with $K-1$ degrees of freedom. If $\mathbf{S}_w' \mathbf{V}_w^{-1} \mathbf{S}_w$ exceeds that value, then reject the null hypothesis of equivalent survival in the K groups in favor of the alternative that their survival distributions differ. As an alternative, find the probability that a random variable that has a χ^2 distribution with $K-1$ degrees of freedom has a value that exceeds $\mathbf{S}_w' \mathbf{V}_w^{-1} \mathbf{S}_w$. This is the p-value of the test statistic. Reject the null hypothesis if that p-value is less than α.

Of course, the reader of this book undoubtably has access to SAS software and a computer to run it on. Thus, you will not actually be doing the above steps. Nevertheless, it is useful to know how PROC LIFETEST and the macro described below work.

5. Using the LIFETEST Procedure

5.1 The STRATA Statement and the Output It Generates

The LIFETEST procedure can perform the log rank test and the Gehan test (referred to in the output and documentation as the Wilcoxon test) to compare two or more groups with respect to time to death. To get these results, you simply add to the statements that invoke PROC LIFETEST a statement of the form

```
strata varname(s);
```

where each *varname* is the name of a grouping variable, and more than one may be specified. If a numeric variable is used, it may be followed by a list of the form $(a_1, a_2, \ldots, a_m)$. Such a list creates strata of the form $x < a_1, a_1 \le x < a_2, \ldots, a_{m-1} \le x < a_m$, and $a_m \le x$. The output of PROC LIFETEST will then contain

- life tables, as described in Chapter 2, for each combination of strata defined by *varname(s)*.

- plots requested for each combination of strata.

- the vector $\Sigma(\mathbf{d}_i - \mathbf{E}_i)$ of log rank scores and $\Sigma R_i(\mathbf{d}_i - \mathbf{E}_i)$ of Gehan (Wilcoxon) scores as well as their covariance matrices.

- the resultant χ^2 statistics and their *p*-values.

- the asymptotic likelihood ratio test statistic for testing the equality of the hazards of exponential distributions. It is valid only if the survival distributions of each of the groups being compared is exponential. By contrast, the other two statistics and their *p*-values require no distributional assumptions. This statistic and other parametric methods are discussed in Chapter 5.

5.2 An Example

For an example of the use of PROC LIFETEST to compare survival distributions, return to the data from a Pediatric Oncology Group leukemia study that was used in Chapter 2, and compare that data to that of another treatment group in the same study. Label the previously described group and this new group 1 and 2, respectively. PROC LIFETEST produces Output 3.1 in addition to the life tables for each group (which are omitted here).

Output 3.1

```
                         Comparing Two Groups

                        The LIFETEST Procedure

        Summary of the Number of Censored and Uncensored Values

        GROUP        Total       Failed    Censored   %Censored

        1              65           23          42     64.6154
        2              64           27          37     57.8125


        Total         129           50          79     61.2403

                         Comparing Two Groups

                        The LIFETEST Procedure

          Testing Homogeneity of Survival Curves over Strata
                       Time Variable YEARS

                           Rank Statistics

              GROUP          Log-Rank       Wilcoxon

                1            -2.9533        -263.00
                2          ❶ 2.9533       ❷ 263.00

        Covariance Matrix for the Log-Rank Statistics

              GROUP                1               2

                1              12.4658        -12.4658
                2             -12.4658         12.4658  ❸

        Covariance Matrix for the Wilcoxon Statistics

              GROUP                1               2

                1             121786         -121786
                2            -121786          121786  ❸

               Test of Equality over Strata

                                              Pr >
              Test      Chi-Square    DF    Chi-Square

           Log-Rank       0.6997 ❹     1      0.4029 ❺
           Wilcoxon       0.5680       1      0.4511 ❻
           -2Log(LR)      0.5894       1      0.4427
```

From this output you can surmise the following:

❶ There were about three fewer deaths than expected under the null hypothesis in group 1 and, of course, about three more than expected in group 2.

❷ When the differences of the numbers of deaths at each time from that expected are weighted by the numbers at risk and summed over all death times, those weighted sums are -263 and 263 for groups 1 and 2, respectively.

❸ The variances of these sums are 12.46548 and 121786 for the log rank and Gehan sums, respectively.

❹ The values of the χ^2 statistics for these two tests are $2.9533^2/12.46548 = 0.6997$ for the log rank test and $263^2/121786 = 0.5680$ for the Gehan test.

❺ Both tests fail to offer any evidence that the two treatments differ with respect to time to death. The p-values are 0.4029 for the log rank test and 0.4511 for the Gehan test.

5.3 A Word of Caution

In this case, both tests yield the same conclusion; however, this may not always be true. In fact, Prentice and Marek (1979) give an interesting example, based on real data, in which the p-value for the log rank test was 0.01, but the p-value for the Gehan test was 0.76! It is important to specify in advance the statistical test to be used and to honor that choice when the analyses are done. Later in this chapter, you will learn how power considerations may provide a reason for a preference. Unless you have such a reason for a preference, you should probably use the log rank test.

6. A Test for Trend

In some cases you might find it reasonable to assume that the difference between groups, if any, should be in a certain direction. For example, the groups might be determined by the extent of disease. Groups 1, 2, and 3 can represent increasing extents. Then, if these groups do differ in survival, you would expect to find not simply a difference in the components of $\Sigma w_i(\mathbf{d}_i - \mathbf{E}_i)$ but also to find that those components are in ascending order. Similarly, if higher numbered groups are defined by increasing doses of a drug that you believe is beneficial, and if increasing doses are associated with increased benefit, you would expect the components of $\Sigma w_i(\mathbf{d}_i - \mathbf{E}_i)$ to be decreasing. Since, for a given sample, a test of a null hypothesis against a specific ordered alternative has greater power than does an omnibus test against any alternative, in cases such as those discussed earlier in this section, you might want to test for a trend. If each group j is associated with a quantitative variable such as drug dose, x_j, let $\mathbf{x}$ be the column vector $(x_1, x_2, \ldots, x_K)'$. The scalar $\mathbf{x}'\Sigma w_i(\mathbf{d}_i - \mathbf{E}_i)\mathbf{x}$ can be considered to be normally distributed. Under the null hypothesis of equivalent survival, its mean is 0 and its variance is the scalar $\mathbf{x}'\mathbf{Cx}$ where $\mathbf{C}$ is the covariance matrix of $\Sigma w_i(\mathbf{d}_i - \mathbf{E}_i)$. Thus you can compare $[\mathbf{x}'\Sigma w_i(\mathbf{d}_i - \mathbf{E}_i)\mathbf{x}]^2/[\mathbf{x}'\mathbf{Cx}]$ to the appropriate critical value from a χ^2 distribution with 1 degree of freedom. If the groups have a natural ordering that is not associated with a quantity, you can replace the vector **x** with $(1, 2, \ldots, K)'$. You might do this, for example, to compare groups with stage II, III, and IV breast cancer. An example is given later in this chapter in "The Macro LINRANK."

7. Stratified Analyses

7.1 The Idea of Stratification

If the groups you are comparing are created by randomizing patients to different treatment regimens, then they probably will be roughly equivalent with respect to other factors which might influence survival, such as age, sex, and severity of disease. Factors that influence survival are said to be prognostic for survival. You might force the treatment groups to be equivalent with respect to some prognostic factor by the manner in which you set up the treatment assignment. For example, if you want to compare two treatments and you feel that males and females have different survival rates, then you can randomize males and females separately in blocks of four so that each block of four patients of the same sex has two on each treatment. Thus, both treatment groups will have about the same proportion of males. If, however, you are comparing patients in naturally occurring groups, such as race, sex, tumor histology and so on, then these groups may very well differ in the distribution of some other factor that is prognostic for survival.

For example, in a study of neuroblastoma, investigators with the Pediatric Oncology Group (POG) noticed that children with diploid tumors seemed to have worse survival than did those whose tumors were hyperdiploid (Look et al. 1991). It was also noticed that those with diploid tumors tended to have more advanced disease (described by POG staging criteria as stage A, B, C, or D) than did those with hyperdiploid tumors. The investigators were interested in whether the prognostic effect of ploidy was due to its association with more advanced disease or whether ploidy is prognostic for survival independent of disease stage. They compared children with diploid tumors to those with hyperdiploid tumors by doing log rank tests that were stratified by other known prognostic factors such as stage and age. Thus, they were able to establish that tumor ploidy is an important prognostic factor independent of these other prognostic factors. As a result of these analyses, in subsequent treatment studies of this disease by the POG, children with diploid tumors were given more intensive treatment (Bowman et al., in press).

7.2 The Stratified Statistic

To perform any of the linear rank tests described earlier in this chapter with stratification by a variable that takes on Q values, say $1, 2, \ldots, Q$, begin by computing the vector of weighted differences and the covariance matrix of that difference for each of the Q strata. Denote by $\mathbf{S}_{wq}$ and $\mathbf{V}_{wq}$ the vector of differences and its covariance matrix for stratum q. As in Section 3, each $\mathbf{S}_{wq}$ must have one component deleted and each $\mathbf{V}_{wq}$ must have that corresponding row and column deleted. Then $(\Sigma \mathbf{S}_{wq})'(\Sigma \mathbf{V}_{wq})^{-1}(\Sigma \mathbf{S}_{wq})$ has, under the null hypothesis, a χ^2 distribution. Here the indicated sums are over $q = 1, 2, \ldots Q$. The number of degrees of freedom is the dimension of each $\mathbf{S}_{wq}$, namely one less than the number of groups being compared. Of course, for each q, $\mathbf{S}'_{wq} \mathbf{V}_w{}^{-1} \mathbf{S}_{wq}$ provides a test statistic for the comparison of the groups in stratum q.

8. The Macro LINRANK

8.1 LINRANK's Capabilities

The macro LINRANK provides several more capabilities than does PROC LIFETEST. For example, it allows the user to specify any one of a broader range of linear rank tests. In addition to the log rank and Gehan (Wilcoxon) tests, those proposed by Tarone and Ware (1977) and by Harrington and Fleming (1982) can also be performed. Recall that the Harrington and Fleming weights are formed by raising an estimated survival function to a power, ρ. In this case, the left-continuous Kaplan-Meier estimator (discussed earlier in Section 4.2) is used, and the exponent, ρ, can also be specified. A value of -1 gives the statistic of Gray and Tsiatis. If the Harrington and Fleming weights are chosen, the default value of ρ is 1. The default is the log rank test. Stratification is permitted, and the test for trend is done if there are more than two groups being compared. If there are $K > 2$ groups, then the default group weights are $(1, 2, \ldots, K)$ where the j'th group in the natural ordering of the group names is assigned weight j. Optionally, if the group names are numeric, drug dosage, for example, the user can specify that the group names are to be the group weights in the trend test. Finally, the output includes the numbers and expected numbers of deaths in each group as well as the value of χ^2 and the associated p-value. If a stratified analysis is requested, then stratum results as well as well as pooled results are given. Because matrix operations are needed in the calculation of the test statistics, PROC IML is used. The macro listing is given at the end of this chapter.

The use of this macro can be facilitated by using the following template and filling in values for the parameters.

```
%linrank(
          dataset=            /* default is _last_ */
         ,time=               /* name of time variable, default is
                              time */
         ,event=              /* name of event variable */
         ,censval=            /* value(s) of event variable that
                              indicate censoring */
         ,groupvar=           /* name of grouping variable */
         ,method=             /* test to be done - choices are
                                 log rank (default)
                                 gehan
                                 tarone
                                 harrington  */

         ,rho=                /* exponent used with harrington test
                               - default is 1, -1 gives the
                              Gray/Tsiatis statistic */
         ,stratvar=           /* name of stratification variable -
                               default is _none_ */
         ,stratmis=           /* use yes for counting missing value
                                for stratvar as a stratum -
                              default is no */
         ,trend=              /* use order (default) to cause group
                                weights for trend test to be
                                determined by natural order of the
                                group names - values for group
                                names (numeric) to be weights */

        )
```

8.2 An Example (Unstratified)

As an example of the use of this macro, consider some breast cancer data from the cancer registry maintained by the H. Lee Moffitt Cancer Center and Research Institute. In addition to survival data, that registry also contains the patient's age at diagnosis, stage of disease, and many other variables. For purposes of this analysis, age at diagnosis will be classified as 0—59, 60—69, 70—79, or 80+. Of course, other breakdowns of this variable are possible and could lead to different results. In Chapters 4 and 5 you will learn about methods to analyze the effect of a continuous variables such as age on survival. First, do an unstratified analysis comparing the age groups. For this analysis, the default log rank test was used. The following code invokes the macro LINRANK:

```
%linrank(
        time=years        /* name of time variable, default is
                             time */
      ,event= cens        /* name of event variable */
      ,censval= 0         /* value(s) of event variable that
                             indicate censoring */
      ,groupvar= agegrp   /* name of grouping variable */
)
```

The results are given as Output 3.2.

Output 3.2

```
                    Summary of Events vs Expected

                        Method = logrank


                  Percent of                              ❶  ❷
         Frequency    Total                            Weighted
AGEGRP     Count   Frequency Events Expected    Diff      Diff

0-59        891    56.2855     157   133.468  23.5322   23.5322
60-69       404    25.5212      46    72.174 -26.1743  -26.1743
70-79       217    13.7081      25    34.400  -9.3999   -9.3999
80+          71     4.4852      20     7.958  12.0420   12.0420
         =========                 ======
            1583                     248


                     Covariance Matrix

                     Method = logrank


     AGEGRP       0-59        60-69       70-79         80+


       0-59     61.3591    -38.5470    -18.4795     -4.33263
      60-69    -38.5470     50.8465    -10.0396     -2.25993
      70-79    -18.4795    -10.0396     29.6144     -1.09533
       80+      -4.3326     -2.2599     -1.0953      7.68790
```

```
                        Method = logrank
                              ❸
        RESULTS CHISQUARE          DF   P_VALUE

              34.661396           3 1.4364E-7


        TREND CHISQUARE           DF   P_VALUE

              2.5572587           1 0.1097888
```

The results in Output 3.2 offer strong evidence that the patient's age is an important factor in survival. Note the following features of this output:

❶ Because the log rank test was performed, the last column of the Summary of Events vs Expected table is the same as the column preceding it. If any other test had been specified, they would differ.

❷ A negative value in the final column of the Summary of Events vs Expected table indicates a group with better than expected survival. A positive value indicates a group with worse than expected survival. In this case, the results indicate that the youngest (0–59 years old) and oldest women (80+ years old) with breast cancer did worse than those of intermediate (60–79) ages.

❸ The test is highly significant for the comparison of the age groups. The test for trend was not significant. This is not surprising considering the observation in this list's second item. The values in the Diff column were not uniformly increasing or decreasing.

Note that the natural order of the group names is from youngest to oldest. Thus, the trend test assigned group weights in that order. If you wanted to test for a different trend, you would need to rename the groups accordingly.

8.3 Continuing the Example (Stratified)

It has been suggested that the poor survival among the younger women may be accounted for by the fact that they tend to have more advanced disease when diagnosed. In fact, for this data, 19.5% of the women in the 0–59 year old group were diagnosed with stage III or IV disease compared to 9.0% of the older women. Thus, you can next consider the effect of redoing the analysis, stratifying on stage. Adding STRATVAR=STAGE to the macro invocation produces a list of deleted observations and a Summary of Events vs Expected for each value of STAGE, as shown in Output 3.3.

Output 3.3

```
                          Deleted Observations  ❶

      OBS       OBSNUMB       YEARS        CENS       AGEGRP       STAGE

       1          309        2.26146        0         0-59
       2          426        7.04997        0         0-59
       3          508        0.34497        0         0-59
       4          510        8.30938        0         0-59
       5          675        0.42163        0         0-59
       6         1223        0.02738        0         60-69
       7         1236        2.20945        0         60-69
       8         1312        3.58385        0         70-79
       9         1373        2.36277        0         70-79
      10         1425        0.00000        0         70-79
      11         1430        0.01643        0         70-79
      12         1452        4.30664        0         70-79
      13         1494        0.15332        0         70-79
      14         1563        0.45175        1         80+
      15         1565        1.49760        1         80+
      16         1575        0.04654        0         80+


                        Summary of Events vs Expected
                                 stage = 0
                             Method = logrank


                      Percent of
            Frequency    Total                             Weighted
   AGEGRP     Count    Frequency  Events  Expected   Diff     Diff

   0-59         91     48.6631       1    1.91586 -0.91586 -0.91586
   60-69        57     30.4813       2    1.13006  0.86994  0.86994
   70-79        31     16.5775       1    0.84618  0.15382  0.15382
   80+           8      4.2781       0    0.10789 -0.10789 -0.10789
              =========             ======
                187                    4


                          Covariance Matrix
                               stage = 0
                           Method = logrank
      AGEGRP        0-59         60-69        70-79         80+

      0-59        0.99356      -0.54020     -0.40138     -0.05197
      60-69      -0.54020       0.81050     -0.23983     -0.03047
      70-79      -0.40138      -0.23983      0.66367     -0.02246
      80+        -0.05197      -0.03047     -0.02246      0.10491
```

```
                        stage = 0
                    Method = logrank


         RESULTS CHISQUARE           DF   P_VALUE

                   1.2469267          3 0.7417727


         TREND CHISQUARE             DF   P_VALUE

                   0.4481371          1   0.503221
```

```
                 Summary of Events vs Expected
                          stage = I
                      Method = logrank

                     Percent of
           Frequency   Total                         Weighted
AGEGRP       Count   Frequency Events Expected  Diff    Diff

0-59          278     47.6844    13    16.1789 -3.17887 -3.17887
60-69         179     30.7033     7    12.3430 -5.34299 -5.34299
70-79          96     16.4666     5     5.6261 -0.62613 -0.62613
80+            30      5.1458    10     0.8520  9.14799  9.14799
           =========          ======
              583               35


                    Covariance Matrix
                         stage = I
                     Method = logrank

    AGEGRP       0-59         60-69        70-79        80+

    0-59       8.67900      -5.67309     -2.60603     -0.39988
    60-69     -5.67309       7.93445     -1.97235     -0.28901
    70-79     -2.60603      -1.97235      4.71560     -0.13723
    80+       -0.39988      -0.28901     -0.13723      0.82612


                         stage = I
                     Method = logrank


         RESULTS CHISQUARE           DF   P_VALUE

                   101.91377          3        0


         TREND CHISQUARE             DF   P_VALUE

                   10.344417          1 0.0012987   ❸
```

```
                     Summary of Events vs Expected
                              stage = II
                           Method = logrank


                          Percent of
               Frequency    Total                          Weighted
  AGEGRP        Count     Frequency  Events  Expected   Diff     Diff

  0-59           344      61.1012      63    56.2464   6.75360   6.75360
  60-69          126      22.3801      22    30.3995  -8.39949  -8.39949
  70-79           72      12.7886      11    10.7026   0.29743   0.29743
  80+             21       3.7300       5     3.6515   1.34846   1.34846
              =========              ======
                 563                   101



                           Covariance Matrix
                              stage = II
                           Method = logrank


    AGEGRP        0-59         60-69        70-79         80+

    0-59        24.5870     -16.4823     -6.04941     -2.05526
    60-69      -16.4823      20.6423     -3.09449     -1.06550
    70-79       -6.0494      -3.0945      9.53614     -0.39224
    80+         -2.0553      -1.0655     -0.39224      3.51301



                             stage = II
                           Method = logrank



           RESULTS CHISQUARE        DF    P_VALUE

                 3.7339275           3  0.2916656



           TREND CHISQUARE           DF    P_VALUE

                 0.6864301           1  0.4073813
```

```
                        Summary of Events vs Expected   ❷
                                stage = III
                              Method = logrank


                        Percent of
              Frequency    Total                                    Weighted
   AGEGRP      Count     Frequency  Events  Expected    Diff          Diff

   0-59         119       80.9524     47    44.3302   2.66980       2.66980
   60-69         20       13.6054      5     7.1582  -2.15821      -2.15821
   70-79          4        2.7211      2     2.4610  -0.46102      -0.46102
   80+            4        2.7211      0     0.0506  -0.05057      -0.05057
             =========                   ======
                147                          54


                              Covariance Matrix
                                 stage = III
                              Method = logrank


     AGEGRP       0-59          60-69         70-79          80+

      0-59       7.91722      -5.87139      -2.00434      -0.041479
      60-69     -5.87139       6.19387      -0.31560      -0.006873
      70-79     -2.00434      -0.31560       2.32141      -0.001465
      80+       -0.04148      -0.00687      -0.00146       0.049816


                                stage = III
                              Method = logrank



              RESULTS CHISQUARE          DF    P_VALUE

                    0.9507267            3  0.8131722


              TREND CHISQUARE            DF    P_VALUE

                    0.8189169            1   0.365497
```

```
                    Summary of Events vs Expected
                             stage = IV
                          Method = logrank


                           Percent of
             Frequency        Total                          Weighted
 AGEGRP        Count        Frequency  Events  Expected   Diff    Diff


  0-59          54          62.0690     33    30.1656  2.83445  2.83445
 60-69          20          22.9885     10    12.4233 -2.42330 -2.42330
 70-79           8           9.1954      6     6.1481 -0.14811 -0.14811
 80+             5           5.7471      3     3.2630 -0.26304 -0.26304
             =========                ======
                87                       52



                         Covariance Matrix
                             stage = IV
                          Method = logrank


    AGEGRP         0-59          60-69         70-79          80+


     0-59       12.5412       -7.19399      -3.49115      -1.85609
    60-69       -7.1940        9.34152      -1.41367      -0.73386
    70-79       -3.4912       -1.41367       5.31395      -0.40912
    80+         -1.8561       -0.73386      -0.40912       2.99907



                            stage = IV
                          Method = logrank



  RESULTS CHISQUARE          DF    P_VALUE

         0.7692193            3  0.8568143



  TREND CHISQUARE            DF    P_VALUE

         0.4250801            1   0.514413
```

```
                  Summary of Events vs Expected
                  Pooled Over All Values of stage

                        Percent of                               ❷
           Frequency      Total                               Weighted
  AGEGRP     Count      Frequency  Events  Expected    Diff     Diff

   0-59       886       56.5412     157   148.837    8.1631    8.1631
  60-69       402       25.6541      46    63.454  -17.4541  -17.4541
  70-79       211       13.4652      25    25.784   -0.7840   -0.7840
  80+          68        4.3395      18     7.925   10.0749   10.0749
           =========                    ======
              1567                        246


                     Covariance Matrix
                 Pooled Over All Values of stage

    AGEGRP        0-59          60-69         70-79         80+

     0-59        54.7180      -35.7610      -14.5523      -4.40469
    60-69       -35.7610       44.9226       -7.0359      -2.12571
    70-79       -14.5523       -7.0359       22.5508      -0.96252
    80+          -4.4047       -2.1257       -0.9625       7.49292


                      Pooled Results
                     Method = logrank
                                        ❷
          RESULTS CHISQUARE       DF    P_VALUE

              18.523151            3   0.000343


          TREND CHISQUARE          DF    P_VALUE

              0.0255948            1  0.8728938
```

Note the following features of Output 3.3:

❶ For sixteen patients, results for STAGE were missing from the data set. Since this analysis used the default, which does not count missing values as stratum values, those patients are excluded from the analysis and a list of them is printed. If we had specified STRATMISS=YES, these sixteen patients would have been used as another stratum. For the previous, unstratified analysis, all patients had valid values for all needed variables, so no such listing was printed.

❷ In this data set, STAGE apparently accounts for some, but not all, of the age group effect on survival. This can be seen in two ways. First, notice that in the pooled Summary of Events vs Expected, the differences still indicate worse survival for the youngest and oldest patients. Their absolute values are, however, smaller than those of the unstratified table. Second, the pooled results still are highly significant, but with a smaller value of chi-square.

❸   It is interesting to note that for one of the strata, the patients with stage I disease, we do see evidence of diminished survival with greater age. The *p*-value for the trend test is about 0.001. One reason to do a stratified analysis is to determine whether an effect is different in different subgroups.

9. The Mantel-Byar Method

9.1 The Basic Idea of the Mantel-Byar Method

Turn now to a slightly different situation. Consider a cohort of patients who are each, on a certain date, considered candidates for an organ transplant. In general, they will have some waiting time until they can get their transplants. Some will die or be censored without ever getting transplants. Some will die or be censored after receiving the transplant. You would like to analyze the effect of the transplant on survival. Clearly, it will not be very useful to use only the methods described earlier in this chapter and thereby to simply compare the transplanted patients to those not transplanted. Those who died early were likely to have been poor prognosis patients. Since they died early, they probably would be in the untransplanted group. Those who got transplanted had to survive long enough to get one and, thus, might have had better prognoses. There is, however, a simple modification of the log rank test, first presented by Mantel and Byar (1974), that addresses questions of this sort in an appropriate manner. An alternative method of dealing with data of this type will be discussed in Chapter 4, "Proportional Hazards Regression."

Think of the patients as originally being in the pre-transplant state. They may die or be censored while still in this state, or they may receive a transplant, thus changing from the pre-transplant to the post-transplant state. In that state, they may die or be censored. The question then becomes whether the data provide evidence that the two states differ in their impact on survival. In this example (which was the motivation for the paper by Mantel and Byar) there are only two states and only one possible state change. It is not any more difficult to allow much greater generality. Suppose there are K states. For convenience, label them $1, 2, \ldots, K$. The ordering is not important here. Patients enter the study in one of these states. They can each make any number of state changes, from any of the states to any of the others, at any times. Each patient is finally censored or dies in one of the states. This more general formulation of their method was suggested by Mantel and Byar in their paper. Cantor (1994) describes this in greater detail and presents a SAS macro for its implementation.

The essential idea of the Mantel-Byar method is to have a table similar to the one used in the log rank test to keep track of the number at risk and number who die *in each state* at the time of each death. The departure from the log rank test is due to the fact that, in addition to diminishing the number at risk in each state when a patient in that state dies or is censored, you also diminish the number in state j_1 and increase the number in state j_2 when a patient goes from state j_1 to state j_2. Once you change the way the R_{ij} (the number at risk in state j at the time of the i'th death) is calculated, all of the formulas for **d**, **E**, and the variances and covariances of $\mathbf{d} - \mathbf{E}$ in Sections 3.1 and 3.2 hold. Crowley (1974) has shown that the statistic $\mathbf{S'V^{-1}S}$ (which is defined just as it is in that section) has, asymptotically, a χ^2 distribution with $K-1$ degrees of freedom under the null hypothesis of equivalent survival in each state, just as the log rank statistic does.

9.2 The MANTBYAR Macro

9.2.1 Organization of the Data Set

In order to permit the flexibility of state changes as described in the previous section, it is necessary to use a slightly more complex method of describing the data to be analyzed. First of all, there must be a variable that serves as a unique identifier for each patient. The name of this variable is specified in the macro call, but will be ID in this description. Two other variables, which are called STATE and TIME here, are also used. Each observation tells the macro that a patient identified by ID entered the state identified by STATE at time TIME. TIME is 0 for an observation that indicates a patient's entry onto the study. If there are K states, they are labeled $1, 2, \ldots, K$. A patient who is censored is thought of as entering state 0. A patient who dies is thought of as entering state $K + 1$. For example, suppose a patient with ID = 1 starts in a study by entering in state 3. He changes to state 1 at time 34, to state 4 at time 40, and back to state 3 at time 51. Finally, he is censored while in state 3 at time 65. The part of the data set based on this patient looks like Table 3.3.

Table 3.3

ID	STATE	TIME
1	3	0
1	1	34
1	4	40
1	3	51
1	0	65

Of course, there will be similar observations for each of the other patients. The observations do not have to be sorted by ID or TIME.

9.2.2 Invoking the Macro

The MANTBYAR macro is invoked by a macro call which sets values for the macro variables that give the name of the SAS data set to be used; the names of the identifier, state, and time variables; the number of states and, optionally, a format for the state variable. The default data set is the last data set defined, the default identifier variable is ID, the default time variable is TIME, and the default number of states is 2. The default format for the state variable is to associate the format STATE1 with 1, STATE2 with 2, and so on. The macro can be invoked by filling the spaces in the following template.

```
%macro mantbyar(
dataset =                    /* default is _last_ */
,state =                     /* name of the state variable */
,time =                      /* name of time variable, default is
                                time */
,nstates =                   /* the number states, default is 2 */
,format =                    /* format for state variable, default
                                is STATE1, STATE2, etc*/
,id =                        /* the unique patient identifier,
                                default is id */

)
```

The output produced by this macro contains the covariance matrix for testing the O– E's for each state and a table of observed and expected number of events in each state with a *p*-value for the association of each state with the event. Each of these *p*-values is based on comparing the O–E divided by its standard deviation to the standard normal distribution. Finally, an overall test of the homogeneity of the states is given. This is based on comparing the statistic $\mathbf{S'V^{-1}S}$ to a χ^2 distribution with $K-1$ degrees of freedom.

9.2.3 An Example

The Natural History of Insulin Dependent Diabetes Mellitus (IDDM) is a study that created and maintains a database of siblings of children with IDDM (Riley et al. 1990). At the time of the analysis described in this section, there were 1354 children in the database. All were non-diabetic upon entry. One of the study's objectives was to follow these children for conversion to IDDM and to look for factors related to conversion. One of the factors that was studied is the level of insulin antibodies as measured in JDF units. At any time, a patient is classified into one of five states as follows:

Antibody Level (JDF units)	State
< 20	1
≥ 20, < 40	2
≥ 40, < 80	3
≥ 80, < 160	4
≥ 160	5

The results of running the MANTBYAR macro with this data are given in Output 3.4.

Output 3.4

```
                          Covariance Matrix

COV         STATE1      STATE2      STATE3      STATE4      STATE5

STATE1      1.0016     -0.2645     -0.2063     -0.2879     -0.2429
STATE2     -0.2645      0.2704     -0.0018     -0.0025     -0.0016
STATE3     -0.2063     -0.0018      0.2113     -0.0021     -0.0011
STATE4     -.02879     -0.0025     -0.0021      0.2941     -0.0021
STATE5     -0.2429     -0.0016     -0.0011     -0.0016      0.2472


                 Summary of Results for Each State

STATE     Observed      Expected          O/E      O-E ❶    P-Value❷

STATE1     11.0000       32.9656       0.3337    -21.965      0.0000
STATE2      3.0000        0.2728      10.9990      2.7272      0.0000
STATE3      4.0000        0.2130      18.7820      3.7870      0.0000
STATE4     12.0000        0.2971      40.3921     11.7029      0.0000
STATE5      4.0000        0.2516      15.8984      3.7484      0.0000

                 Test of Homogeneity of States ❸

            CHISQ                  DF                   P

           626.7672                4                 0.0000
```

❶   The O-E column shows the impact of each state on the occurrence of the endpoint (in this case conversion to IDDM). The negative value for STATE1 and the positive values for the other states show that STATE1 (antibody level < 20) had fewer conversions and that the other states had more conversions than would be expected if all states carried equivalent conversion risk.

❷   The P-Value column gives the *p*-value for the effect of each state. In this case, each one is significant. Of course, the *p*-values are not truly 0.0000. This value is printed because each is less than 0.00001.

❸   The Test of Homogeneity of States is a test of the null hypothesis that there is no difference in states versus the alternative that there is <u>some</u> difference. Not suprisingly, this is highly significant as well.

A listing of the MANTBYAR macro is given at the end of this chapter.

10. Power Analysis

10.1 Introduction

In most areas of statistics, given a study design, significance level, and values for the population parameters, the power of the test to be done can be shown to be a function of the sample size. By "solving for the sample size," or perhaps by performing some crude iteration, you can determine the sample size that will produce the desired power (often 80% or 90%). Lachin (1981) provides an excellent introduction to this subject. In survival analysis, however, the situation is quite different. This is because the amount of information about survival conveyed by a sample is not determined by the sample size alone, but also by the amount of time those in the sample have been observed. Thus, the following features of a study have to be considered in discussing its power:

1.   the significance level of the test to be done.

2.   the length of the accrual period.

3.   the amount of post-accrual follow-up time.

4.   the accrual rate. This is the rate at which patients are entered onto the study.

5.   the distribution(s) of the loss to follow-up.

6.   the survival distributions of the groups being compared.

The first three of these are under your control as the study planner. The last three are generally not subject to your control, although in some cases you can impact on the accrual rate by the effort and resources devoted to accrual or by the number of institutions that are asked to participate in a multi-institutional study. Similarly, loss to follow-up may be, in some cases, affected by the effort taken to reduce it. The survival distributions of the groups being compared must, of course, be hypothesized. They should have some basis in prior experience. Also, they should be sufficiently different that such a difference would be clinically meaningful, but not so different as to be unrealistic.

In the next section, a power formula for linear rank tests comparing two groups is given. Methods that can be applied to three or more groups have been discussed (Makuch and Simon, 1982, Liu and Dahlberg, 1995), but they are somewhat limited. Their methods require the assumption that the survival distributions being compared are exponential and can deal with the log rank test only. The second of these reports provides a SAS program for calculating the required sample size when comparing four groups using the log rank test.

10.2 The Formula for Power Calculations

In what follows, assume that the study planners have specified items 1 – 6 above, and you wish to estimate the power of certain linear rank tests (including the log rank test and the Gehan test) resulting from those specifications. By perturbing those specifi-cations, you can then, hopefully, determine study parameters that are realistic and that will achieve the desired power. Many approaches to this problem assume that survival distributions of the two groups being compared are exponential (George and Desu, 1974 and Rubenstein, Gail, and Santner, 1981). Others allow for other distributions, but require that the proportional hazard assumption holds (Shuster, 1990 and Cantor, 1992). In these cases, the asymptotic efficiency of the log rank test can be shown to lead to a fairly simple result for the power of that test (Shuster, 1990).

Experience with actual clinical trials suggests, however, that such assumptions are not necessarily realistic. For this reason, the method presented here, which is due to Lakatos (1988), requires no assumption concerning the survival distributions of the groups being compared. His formulation allows for rather complex designs and permits specifying the effects of crossovers and non-compliers. Shih (1995) discusses a program that implements the Lakatos method, maintaining the functionality described by Lakatos. This section presents a SAS macro, SURVPOW, that also implements the Lakatos method. While SURVPOW does not allow for some of the complexity of the Lakatos approach as Shih does, it may be easier for the user to invoke. Because it usually is easier to describe survival distributions of groups being compared in terms of survival probabilities at various times rather than by values of their hazard functions, SURVPOW allows you to specify the alternative distributions in that way. Abandonment of the proportional hazards assumption allows for the possibility that an alternative linear rank test may have greater power than the log rank test. Thus, you may specify a large class of such alternative test statistics.

Suppose you plan to accrue patients to a clinical trial that is designed to compare two groups, for T units of time at rate r per time unit. After accrual ends, you will follow the study patients for an additional τ units of time before performing the final analyses. For the purposes of this study, denote the two groups by 1 and 2. To allow for unequal sample sizes, let p be the proportion that you plan to assign to group 1. Then, the sample sizes, N_1 and N_2, are rTp and $rT(1-p)$ respectively. Let $h_j(t)$ be the hazard function, and let $\Psi_j(t)$ be the "hazard" function for patients' being lost to follow-up for group j where $j = 1, 2$.

Now, suppose that the study period $[0, T + \tau]$ is partitioned into subintervals of equal length by $0 = t_0 < t_1 < t_2 < \ldots < t_M = T + \tau$, and let Δ be the common subinterval width. You need to discuss the expected number at risk in each group at each time t_i for the planned study, which is denoted by $N_j(i)$. For each subinterval $[t_i, t_{i+1}]$, the probability of death for a subject in group j can be approximated by $h_j(t_i)\Delta$. Similarly, the probability that this subject will be lost to follow-up in this subinterval is approximately $\Psi_j(t_i)\Delta$. Such subjects are also censored in this subinterval if they entered the study between t_i and t_{i+1} time units prior to $T + \tau$. Assuming uniform accrual, that probability is approximately

$\Delta/(T + \tau - t_i)$ for $t_i > \tau$ and 0 for $t_i \leq \tau$. These considerations lead to the recurrence relation

$$N_j(0) = N_j$$
$$N_j(i + 1) = N_j(i)[1 - h_j(t_i)\Delta - \psi_j(t_i)\Delta] \quad \text{for } t_i \leq \tau$$
$$N_j(i + 1) = N_j(i)\left[1 - h_j(t_i)\Delta - \psi_j(t_i)\Delta - \frac{\Delta}{T + \tau - t_i}\right] \quad \text{for } t_i > \tau \tag{5}$$

Now let $\theta_i = h_1(t_i)/h_2(t_i)$ and $\phi_i = N_1(i)/N_2(i)$. The test statistic given in section 5 by $S_w'V_w^{-1}S_w$ as having a χ^2 distribution with 1 degree of freedom for two groups is a product of scalars in that case. The test is equivalent to comparing $S_w/V_w^{1/2}$ to a critical value of a standard normal distribution. Lakatos shows that this statistic has, in general, a normal distribution with unit variance and mean approximately equal to

$$E = \frac{\sum_{i=1}^{M} D_i w_i \left[\dfrac{\phi_i \theta_i}{1 + \phi_i \theta_i} - \dfrac{\phi_i}{1 + \phi_i}\right]}{\sqrt{\sum_{i=1}^{M} D_i w_i^2 \dfrac{\phi_i}{(1 + \phi_i)^2}}} \tag{6}$$

where $D_i = [h_1(t_i)N_1 + h_2(t_i)N_2]\Delta$, the expected number of deaths in the i'th subinterval. It follows that, for a test being done with significance level α, the power is 1 minus the probability of a standard normal random variable being between $-E - z_{\alpha/2}$ and $-E + z_{\alpha/2}$ where $z_{\alpha/2}$ is the $(1-\alpha/2)100$th percentile of a standard normal distribution.

10.3 The SURVPOW Macro

10.3.1 The Macro's Parameters

The SURVPOW macro takes the following parameters:

S1=
S2=   These are the names of data sets that describe the survival distributions in groups 1 and 2, respectively. They must contain the two variables t (for time) and s (for survival probability at time t). If a data set contains only one observation, (t, s), the macro assumes that the group has exponential survival with $S(t) = s$. This equation determines the constant hazard for that group. If a data set contains exactly two observations and the variable t for the second observation is missing (i.e., has the value '.'), then the "cure" model $S(t) = \pi + (1 - \pi)\exp(-\lambda t)$ is assumed with π being equal to the value of s for the second observation and the first pair (t, s) being a point on the survival

curve. Otherwise, it is assumed that the survival curve is given by the piecewise linear curve that is formed by connecting the points (t, s) for each observation. The values of t and s must satisfy the following conditions:

a. For the first observation, $t = 0$ and $s = 1$.

b. The values of t must be increasing.

c. The values of s must be decreasing.

d. The last value of t must be at least the total time of the study (the accrual time plus the follow-up time).

NSUB=   This is the number of subintervals per time unit. The default is 365, which corresponds to subintervals of one day's duration when the time unit is years.

ACTIME=   This is the number of time units of accrual. It is assumed that accrual occurs uniformly during this interval.

FUTIME=   This is the number of time units for post-accrual follow-up.

RATE=   This is the accrual rate per unit of time.

P=   This is the proportion of patients assigned to group 1. The default is 0.5.

LOSS1=   These are the rates for the assumed loss to follow-up. It is
LOSS2=   assumed that loss to follow-up is exponential. The defaults are 0.

W=   This is the formula for the weights that define the linear rank test that is planned. The variable n, representing the total number at risk, may be used. Thus, $w = 1$ gives the log rank test statistic (the default), $w = n$ gives the Gehan test statistic, and $w = (n**.5)$ gives the test statistic discussed by Tarone and Ware (1977). The parentheses are needed in the last example to assure that the expression $w**2$ is evaluated as intended. That's because SAS will evaluate $n**.5**2$ as $n**.25$ instead of n.

SIGLEVEL=   The (two-sided) significance level for the planned test. The default value is 0.05.

The complete SURVPOW macro is given at the end of this chapter.

This macro can be implemented by filling in values for the parameters in the following template:

```
%survpow(s1=        /* data sets that define the alternative    */
        ,s2=        /* survival distributions for groups 1 and 2*/
        ,nsub=      /* number of subintervals per time unit.
                     Default is 365 */
        ,actime=    /* accrual time */
        ,futime=    /* post-accrual follow-up time   */
        ,rate=      /* accrual rate */
        ,p=         /* proportion assigned to group 1.
                     Default is .5 */
        ,loss1=     /* exponential loss rates in groups 1 and 2.
        ,loss2=     /* Defaults are 0 */
        ,w=         /* weight function. Default is 1 for log rank
                     test. */
        ,siglevel=  /* significant level. Default is 0.05     */
)
```

10.3.2. An Example

As an example, suppose that a clinical trial is being planned to compare a new treatment for Stage IV prostate cancer to a standard treatment. Several hospitals, each able to place 10—20 subjects per year on such a study, are potential participants. The hospitals' experience with the standard treatment can be summarized by a Kaplan-Meier survival curve. Although the entire life table produced by PROC LIFETEST or the LIFETABLE macro could be used as one of the data sets, it is sufficient to use the following yearly survival probability estimates:

Table 3.4

t	$S(t)$
0	1.00
1	0.86
2	0.68
3	0.60
4	0.51
5	0.39
6	0.25
7	0.24
8	0.23

Recall that the values of s must be strictly decreasing. Thus, if there were no deaths after six years (in the sample used to describe survival distribution in one of the study groups) so that s was constant after six years, you would need to create slight annual decreases to use this macro.

Now suppose that the planners don't expect the new treatment to produce much better long term survival, but have reason to believe that it may delay death somewhat. Specifically, they feel that it might have a survival distribution similar to that summarized in the following table.

Table 3.5

t	$S(t)$
0	1.00
1	0.95
2	0.85
3	0.75
4	0.65
7	0.25
8	0.24

To test the null hypothesis of equivalence of the survival distributions for the two treatment groups, use the log rank test with a significance level of 0.05. Half will be assigned to each treatment. Suppose further that there might be little or no loss to follow-up. To start, consider accruing 30 patients per year for four years followed by three years of additional follow-up. The power for this study is estimated by invoking the POWER macro, as shown in the following example:

Example 3.6

```
data group1;
     input t s;
cards;
0               1.00
1               0.86
2               0.68
3               0.60
4               0.51
5               0.39
6               0.25
7               0.24
8               0.23
;
```

```
data group2;
        input t s;
cards;
0                1.00
1                0.95
2                0.85
3                0.75
4                0.65
7                0.25
8                0.24
;
%power(s1=group1   /* data sets that define the alternative */
      ,s2=group2   /* survival distributions for groups 1 and 2*/
      ,actime=4    /* accrual time */
      ,futime=3    /* post-accrual follow-up time   */
      ,rate=30     /* accrual rate */
) ;
```

Note that default values are used for LOSS1, LOSS2, NSUB, SIGLEVEL, P, and W. The results are given in Output 3.6.

Output 3.6

Accrual Time	Follow-up Time	Accrual Rate	N	ALPHA	Prop in Grp 1
4	3	30	120	.05	.5

Loss Rate 1	Loss Rate 2	Weights	Power
0	0	1	0.39087

Clearly this power is inadequate. You would like to have at least an 80% probability of rejecting the null hypothesis if this example's alternative holds. Thus, you need to increase the accrual time, follow-up time, or accrual rate. Of course, the last of these requires getting more institutions to participate. Also, it is possible that, for this example's alternative, another linear rank test may have greater power than the log rank test. If so, that test would be your choice.

The following SAS program shows how the POWER macro may be imbedded in a macro loop in order to consider the power of alternative tests over a range of study parameters. You will consider accrual rates of 40, 45, . . . , 70 per year, and the log rank test, the Gehan test, and the Tarone Ware statistic based on weights equal to the square root of the number at risk. Example 3.7 gives the necessary SAS statements. You need to be familiar with the SAS macro language to understand it.

Example 3.7

```
/* Create data set for weight functions:  n**.5 for the Tarone Ware
statistic, n for the Gehan statistic, and 1 for the log rank
statistic
*/

data data;
    input w $;
cards;
(n**.5)
n
1
;
```

```
/* Create macro variables from weight functions */

data _null_;
      set data;
      i=_n_;
      call symput('w'||left(i), w);
run;

/* Create data sets for alternative */
data group1;
      input t s; cards;
0             1.00
1             0.86
2             0.68
3             0.60
4             0.51
5             0.39
6             0.25
7             0.24
8             0.23
;
data group2;
      input t s;
cards;
0             1.00
1             0.95
2             0.85
3             0.75
4             0.65
7             0.25
8             0.24
;

/* loop on accrual rates and weight functions */

%macro loop;
%do arate=40 %to 70 %by 5;
      %do jj=1 %to 3;
            %power(s1=group1 , s2= group2   ,   actime=4,futime=3
                        ,rate=&arate,w=&&w&jj ) ;
      %end;
%end;
%mend;
%loop;
run;
```

Running this program produces the desired results for three sets of weights and over a range of accrual rates. Only the results for accrual rates of 60 and 65 patients per year are printed in Output 3.7:

Output 3.7

```
                        Power Analysis

   Accrual    Follow-up    Accrual                      Prop in
    Time        Time         Rate       N     ALPHA     Grp 1

      4          3           60        240     .05        .5


   Loss       Loss
  Rate 1     Rate 2     Weights      Power

     0          0        (n**.5)     0.76418
```

```
                           Power Analysis

    Accrual      Follow-up     Accrual                       Prop in
     Time          Time         Rate        N      ALPHA     Grp 1

       4            3            60         240      .05       .5

    Loss         Loss
   Rate 1       Rate 2       Weights       Power

     0            0             n         0.80272


                           Power Analysis

    Accrual      Follow-up     Accrual                       Prop in
     Time          Time         Rate        N      ALPHA     Grp 1

       4            3            60         240      .05       .5

    Loss         Loss
   Rate 1       Rate 2       Weights       Power

     0            0             1         0.66260


                           Power Analyis

    Accrual      Follow-up     Accrual                       Prop in
     Time          Time         Rate        N      ALPHA     Grp 1

       4            3            65         260      .05       .5

    Loss         Loss
   Rate 1       Rate 2       Weights       Power

     0            0          (n**.5)      0.79652


                           Power Analysis

    Accrual      Follow-up     Accrual                       Prop in
     Time          Time         Rate        N      ALPHA     Grp 1
       4            3            65         260      .05       .5

    Loss         Loss
   Rate 1       Rate 2       Weights       Power

     0            0             n         0.83303


                           Power Analysis

    Accrual      Follow-up     Accrual                       Prop in
     Time          Time         Rate        N      ALPHA     Grp 1

       4            3            65         260      .05       .5

    Loss         Loss
   Rate 1       Rate 2       Weights       Power

     0            0             1         0.69732
```

Output 3.7 shows that an accrual rate of 60/year will be sufficient to achieve a power of 80%. That power is achieved for the Gehan test (WEIGHTS = n), but not the log rank test (WEIGHTS = 1). Recall that the Gehan test statistic puts greater weights on earlier deaths, when the number at risk is greater, while the log rank weights are constant. Therefore, for an alternative in which the difference between the two groups being compared is mostly in the early results, as in the previous example, you would expect the Gehan test to have greater power. Note that the Tarone-Ware weights, $n^{1/2}$, which are intermediate between those of the Gehan and the log rank statistic, produce powers intermediate between them as well.

When planning a clinical trial, it is quite common to use a method of power calculation that is based on the assumption of proportional hazards, assuming that the log rank test (which is most powerful in that situation) is to be used to compare the groups. There is considerable literature discussing ways to do this (George and Desu, 1974; Rubenstein, Gail, and Santner, 1981) and, in many cases, such an approach may be appropriate. However, if the planners have some idea of the nature of the alternative that they expect, and if the alternative hazards do not have a constant ratio, then the method described here can be used. The reader is reminded that it is not statistically valid to perform a number of tests on a set of data and then to choose for presentation the result that has the smallest p-value. However, it is quite appropriate, when planning a study, to consider the power of a variety of test statistics for the study parameters and the alternative survival distributions being considered, and then to choose the test with the best power characteristics. Of course, the statistical test to be used should be specified in the study protocol before the study is begun.

11. Complete Macros

11.1. The LINRANK Macro

```
%macro linrank(dataset=_last_, time=time, event=  ,
               censval=   ,groupvar= ,method=logrank,rho=1,
               stratvar= _none_, stratmis=no,trend=order );

/*      Delete invalid observations and
        print list of observations deleted. */

data xx deleted;
     set &dataset;
     obsnumb = _n_;
     if &time <0  or &groupvar=''   or &event = . then delete=1;
     if "&stratvar" ne "_none_" and  "&stratmis" = "no"
     and  &stratvar = '' then delete =1;
     _none_ = 1;
     if delete=1 then output deleted;
     else output xx;
proc print data=deleted;
     title 'Deleted Observations';
     var  obsnumb &time &event &groupvar
     %if "&stratvar" ne "_none_" %then &stratvar;;
```

```
/*        Determine number of groups, their names,
          and the weights to use for trend test.    */

proc sort data = xx;
        by &groupvar;
data y;
        set xx;
        by &groupvar;
        if first.&groupvar then do;
        n+1;
         call symput('ngrps',left(n));
        end;
run;
data grpnames;
        set y;
        by &groupvar;
        keep &groupvar n;
        if first.&groupvar;
data groupwts;
        set grpnames;
        keep
        %if "&trend" = "order" %then n;
        %else &groupvar;;

/* Find number of strata */

proc sort data=xx;
        by &stratvar;
data xx;
        set xx;
        by &stratvar;
        retain stratn 0 ;
        if first.&stratvar then do;
                stratn+1;
                call symput('stratcnt', left(stratn));
        end;
run;

/*      Start loop on strata          */

%do ii = 1 %to &stratcnt;

/*    Form stratum subset, find number of
      groups, number in each group, and
      group weights in stratum                  */

        data x;
                set xx;
                if stratn = &ii;
                call symput('stratval', &stratvar);
        run;
        proc freq;
                table &groupvar/ noprint out= counts;
        proc sort data=x;
                by &groupvar;
        data x;
                set x;
                by &groupvar;
                retain grpn 0 ;
                if first.&groupvar then do;
                                grpn+1;
                    call symput('grpcount', left(grpn));
                    call symput('grpname'||left(grpn), &groupvar);
                     end;
        run;
        data grpnames;
                set x;
                by &groupvar;
                keep &groupvar grpn;
                if first.&groupvar;
        data grpwts;
                set grpnames;
                keep
                %if "&trend" = "order" %then grpn;
                %else &groupvar;;
```

```
/*    Create table        */

     proc sort data=x;
          by descending &time;
     data y;
          set x;
          keep r1-r&grpcount rtot;
          array r{*} r1-r&grpcount;
          retain r1-r&grpcount rtot 0;
          %let countsq = %eval(&grpcount*&grpcount);
          r{grpn}+1;
          rtot+1;
     data x;
          merge x y;
     proc sort;
          by &time;
     data x;
          set x;
          by &time;
          array d{*} d1-d&grpcount;
          retain d1-d&grpcount dtot;
          if first.&time then do i=1 to &grpcount;
               d{i}=0;
               dtot=0;
               end;
          if &event not in (&censval) then do;
               d{grpn}+1;
               dtot+1;
               end;
          if last.&time then output;
     data x;
          set x;
          if dtot>0;
          retain km km_  1;
          all=1;
          array e{*} e1-e&grpcount;
          array diff{*} diff1-diff&grpcount;
          array r{*} r1-r&grpcount;
          array d{*} d1-d&grpcount;
          array wdiff{*} wdiff1-wdiff&grpcount;
          array s{*} sum1-sum&grpcount;
          array cov{&grpcount, &grpcount} cov1-cov&countsq;
          array sumcov{&grpcount,&grpcount}
sumcov1-sumcov&countsq;
          if _n_ = 1 then km_ = 1;
          else km_ = km;
          km=km*(rtot-dtot)/rtot;
          do j=1 to &grpcount;
               e{j} = dtot*r{j}/rtot;
               diff{j} = d{j} - e{j};
               if "&method"="logrank" then w=1;
               if "&method"="gehan" then w=rtot;
               if "&method"="tarone" then w=sqrt(rtot);
               if "&method"="harrington" then w=km_**&rho;
               wdiff{j} = w*diff{j};
               s{j} + wdiff{j};
          do l=1 to &grpcount;
               if dtot=1 then c=1; else
          c=(rtot-dtot)/(rtot-1);
               if j=l then

cov{j,l}=w**2*(dtot*(rtot*r{j}-r{j}**2)*c)/rtot**2;
               else
cov{j,l}=-w**2*(r{j}*r{l}*dtot*c)/rtot**2;
               sumcov{j,l}+cov{j,l};
               end;
          end;
```

```
/*        Sum over times and reformat for printout         */

        proc means sum noprint;
                var d1-d&grpcount e1-e&grpcount diff1-diff&grpcount
                wdiff1-wdiff&grpcount;
                output out = out sum=;
        data out;
        set out;
                array e{*} e1-e&grpcount;
                array d{*} d1-d&grpcount;
                array difff{*} diff1-diff&grpcount;
                array wdif{*} wdiff1-wdiff&grpcount;
                do j = 1 to &grpcount;
                        group = j;
                        events = d{j};
                        expected = e{j};
                        diff = difff{j};
                        wdiff = wdif{j};
                        output;
                        end;
                label wdiff = 'Weighted Diff';
                label events = 'Events';
                label expected = 'Expected';
                label diff = 'Diff';
        data xxx;
                merge out grpnames counts;
        proc print l noobs;
                var &groupvar count percent events expected diff wdiff;
                sum   count events;
                title1 'Summary of Events vs Expected';
                %if "&stratvar" ne "_none_" %then title2 "&stratvar =
                        &stratval";;
                title3 "Method = &method";
        run;

/*        Accumulate vectors and matrices for pooled stats  */

        %if "&ii" = "1" %then %do;
                data pooled;
                        set xxx;
                %end;
        %else %do;
                data pooled;
                set pooled xxx;
                %end;
        data x;
                set x;
        proc sort;
                by all;
        data s (keep = sum1-sum&grpcount) cov (keep =
                        col1-col&grpcount);
                set x;
                by all;
                if last.all;
                array s{*} sum1-sum&grpcount;
                array sumcov{&grpcount, &grpcount}
                        sumcov1-sumcov&countsq;
                array col{*} col1-col&grpcount;
                output s;
                do j=1 to &grpcount;
                        do l=1 to &grpcount;
                        col{l}=sumcov{j,l};
                        end;
                output cov;
                end;
        data yy;
                merge grpnames cov;
```

```
/* Give columns of covariance matrix group names */
        %do j = 1 %to &grpcount;
                label col&j = "&&grpname&j";
                %end;
        proc print 1 noobs;
                var &groupvar col1-col&grpcount;
                title1 'Covariance Matrix';
                %if "&stratvar" ne "_none_" %then title2 "&stratvar=
                        &stratval";;
                title3 "Method = &method";
        %if "&ii" = "1" %then %do;
                data poolcov;
                        set yy;
                %end ;
        %else %do;
                data poolcov;
                set poolcov yy;
                %end;

/*      Use proc iml to do matrix calculations
        for test statistic.                          */

        proc iml;
                reset noprint;
                use s;
                read all into x;
                use cov;
                read all into v;
                use grpwts;
                read all var _all_ into grpwts;

/*      Omit first row and column        */

                xx=x[1:1,2:&grpcount];
                vv=v[2:&grpcount,2:&grpcount];
                stat= xx*inv(vv)*xx`;
                df = &grpcount - 1;
                p_val = 1-probchi(stat,df);
                results = stat||df||p_val;
                cols={ChiSquare df p_value};
                title1 ' ';
                %if "&stratvar" ne "_none_" %then title1 "&stratvar=
                        &stratval";;
                title2 "Method = &method";
                print results[colname=cols];

/*      Test for trend.          */

                if %eval(&grpcount) > 2 then do;
                        wts=grpwts[2:&grpcount, 1:1];
                        xxx=xx*wts;
                        vvv=wts`*vv*wts;
                        stat = xxx*xxx/vvv;
                        df=1;
                        p_val= 1-probchi(stat,df);
                        trend = stat||df||p_val;
                        print trend[colname=cols];
                        end;
                quit;
        %end;

  /* end of loop on strata */

/*      Pooled results if stratified analyis    */

%if "&stratvar" ne "_none_" %then %do;
        proc freq data=xx;
                table &groupvar / noprint out=counts;
        proc sort data=pooled;
                by &groupvar;
        proc means noprint sum data=pooled;
                var count events expected diff wdiff;
                by group;
                output out=pooled1 sum=;
        data;
                merge pooled1 grpnames counts;
```

```
        proc print l noobs;
             var &groupvar count percent events expected diff wdiff;
             sum count events;
             title1 'Summary of Events vs Expected';
             title2 "Pooled Over All Values of &stratvar";
        proc sort data=poolcov;
             by &groupvar;
        proc means noprint sum data=poolcov;
             var col1-col&ngrps;
             by &groupvar;
             output out=pooled2 sum=;
        proc print l noobs;
             var &groupvar col1-col&ngrps;
             title1 'Covariance Matrix';
             title2 "Pooled Over All Values of &stratvar";
        data pooled2;
             set pooled2;
             keep col1-col&ngrps;
        run;
        proc iml;
             reset noprint;
             use pooled1;
             read all var {wdiff} into x;
             use pooled2;
             read all into v;
             xx=x[2:&ngrps,1:1];
             vv=v[2:&ngrps,2:&ngrps];
             stat = xx`*inv(vv)*xx;
             df = &ngrps - 1;
             p_val=1-probchi(stat,df);
             cols={ChiSquare df p_value};
             title1 'Pooled Results';
             title2 "Method = &method";
             results = stat||df|| p_val;
             print results[colname=cols];

  /*      Test for trend.         */

             if %eval(&ngrps) > 2 then do;
                  use groupwts;
                  read all var _all_ into weights;
                  wts = weights[2:&ngrps, 1:1];
                  xtrend = xx`*wts;
                  vtrend = wts`*vv*wts;
                  stattrnd = xtrend**2/vtrend;
                  p_valtrd = 1-probchi(stattrnd,1);
                  df=1;
                  trend=stattrnd||df||p_valtrd;
                  print trend[colname=cols];
                  run;
                  end;
        %end;
%mend;
```

11.2 The SURVPOW Macro

```
%macro survpow(s1=   , s2=    , nsub=365, actime= ,futime=   ,rate=   ,
      p=.5, loss1=0, loss2=0, w=1,siglevel=.05) ;

/* Find number of points in data set for group 1 and convert to
 vectors */

data _null_;
      set &s1;
      i=_n_;
      call symput('counta',left(i));
run;
data y;
      set &s1;
      retain sa1-sa&counta ta1-ta&counta ;
      array surv{*} sa1-sa&counta;
      array ttime{*} ta1-ta&counta;
      t=t*&nsub;
      all=1;
```

```
          i=_n_;
          surv{i}=s;
          ttime{i}=t;
          output;
proc sort;
          by all;
data y;
          set y;
          by all;
          if last.all;
          keep  all ta1-ta&counta sa1-sa&counta;


/*  Find number of points in data set for group 2 and convert to
  vector */


data _null_;
          set &s2;
          i=_n_;
          call symput('countb', left(i));
run;
data yy;
          set &s2;
          retain sb1-sb&countb tb1-tb&countb;
          array surv{*} sb1-sb&countb;
          array ttime{*} tb1-tb&countb;
          t=t*&nsub;
          all=1;
          i=_n_;
          surv{i}=s; ttime{i}=t;
          output;
proc sort;
          by all;
data yy;
          set yy;
          by all;
          if last.all;
          keep  all tb1-tb&countb sb1-sb&countb;


/*  Find hazards at each partition point   */


data z;
          all=1;
          do t=0 to (&actime+&futime)*&nsub;
                    output;
                    end;
proc sort;
          by all;
data merged;
          merge z y yy;
          by all;
          if trim("&counta") = "1" then lam1=-log(sa1)/ta1;
          %do i=1 %to &counta -1 ;
          %let j = %eval(&i+1);
          if ta&i le t lt ta&j then lam1 =
                    (sa&i-sa&j)/((sa&j-sa&i)*(t-ta&i)+sa&i*(ta&j-ta&i));
          %end;
          if trim("&counta") = "2" and ta2 = . then do;
          lambda = -log((sa1-sa2)/(1-sa2))/ta1;
          lam1 = lambda*(1-sa2)*exp(-lambda*t)/
                    (sa2+(1-sa2)*exp(-lambda*t));
          end;
          if trim("&countb") = "1" then lam2=-log(sb1)/tb1;
          %do i=1 %to &countb -1 ;
                    %let j = %eval(&i+1);
                    if tb&i le t lt tb&j then lam2 =
                    (sb&i-sb&j)/((sb&j-sb&i)*(t-tb&i)+sb&i*(tb&j-tb&i));
          %end;
```

```
/*  Calculate ratio of hazards and number at risk at each
    partition point and accumulate needed sums */

data;
        set merged;
        by all;
        retain n1 n2 n;
        if _n_ = 1 then do;
         n1=&rate*&p*&actime;
         n2=&rate*(1-&p)*&actime;
         n=n1+n2;
        end;
        tau=&futime*&nsub;
        psi1=&loss1/&nsub;
        psi2=&loss2/&nsub;
        phi=n1/n2;
        theta=lam1/lam2;
        d1=lam1*n1;
        d2=lam2*n2;
        d=d1+d2;
        c1=psi1*n1;
        c2=psi2*n2;
        if _n_>tau then do;
         c1=c1+n1/(&actime*&nsub+tau-_n_+1);
         c2=c2+n2/(&actime*&nsub+tau-_n_+1);
        end;
        n1=n1-d1-c1;
        n2=n2-d2-c2;
        sum1+(d*&w*(phi*theta/(1+phi*theta)-phi/(1+phi)));
        sum2+d*&w**2*phi/(1+phi)**2;
        n=n1+n2;

/*  Calculate e and power */

        if last.all then do;
                e=sum1/sqrt(sum2);
                z=-probit(&siglevel/2);
                power=1-probnorm(z-e)+probnorm(-z-e);
                ac_time=symget('actime');
                fu_time=symget('futime');
                ac_rate=symget('rate');
                n=ac_rate*ac_time;
                alpha=symget('siglevel');
                prop=symget('p');
                los_rat1=symget('loss1');
                los_rat2=symget('loss2');
                weights=symget('w');
                output;
        end;
        label ac_time='Accrual Time';
        label power='Power';
        label fu_time='Follow-up Time';
        label ac_rate='Accrual Rate';
        label n='N';
        label prop='Prop in Grp 1';
        label los_rat1='Loss Rate 1';
        label los_rat2='Loss Rate 2';
        label weights='Weights';


/*  Print results */

proc print l noobs;
        var ac_time fu_time ac_rate n alpha prop los_rat1 los_rat2
        weights power;
%mend;
```

11.3 The MANTBYAR Macro

```
%macro mantbyar(dataset= last_ , state= , time=time ,nstates=2 ,
                    format= default.,id=id);

/* Create Format for States */

%let form=%str(proc format; value default 1='state1');
%do i=2 %to &nstates;
        %let form=&form &i= %str(%' )STATE&i %str(%');
        %end;
&form;

/* Create Table */

proc sort data= &dataset;
        by &id &time;
data d;
        set &dataset end=last;
        by &id;
        retain id 0;
        if first.&id then id+1;
        if last then call symput('nobs',left(id));
proc sort;
        by &time descending &state;
%let nstat2=%eval(&nstates*&nstates);
%let nm1=%eval(&nstates-1);
data dd;
        set d;
        by &time descending &state;
        retain s1-s&nobs r1-r&nstates o1-o&nstates;
        retain e1-e&nstates 0;
        retain v1-v&nstat2 0;
        retain d1-d&nstates 0;
        array s(*) s1-s&nobs;
        array r(*) r1-r&nstates;
        array e(*) e1-e&nstates;
        array o(*) o1-o&nstates;
        array ot(*) ot1-ot&nstates;
        array v(&nstates,&nstates) v1-v&nstat2;
        array d(*) d1-d&nstates;
        if &time=0 then do;
                s(id)=&state; r(&state)+1;
                nt+1;
                end;
        if &time>0 and &state<&nstates+1 then do;
                prior=s(id);
                r(prior)+(-1);
                if &state>0 then r(&state)+1; s(id)=&state;
                if &state=0 then nt+(-1);
                end;
        if &state=&nstates+1 then do;
                if first.&state then do i=1 to &nstates;
                        ott=0;
                        ot(i)=0;
                        end;
                prior=s(id);
                ot(prior)+1;
                ott+1;

/* Calculate covariance matrix */

        if last.&state then do;
                do i=1 to &nstates;
                        do j= 1 to &nstates;
                        if i=j then v(i,i)+r(i)*(nt-
                        r(i))*ott*(nt-ott)/(nt**2*(nt-1));

                        else v(i,j)+ (-r(i)*r(j)*ott*
                                (nt-ott)/(nt**2*(nt-1)));
                        end;
                end;
```

```
                                                do i=1 to &nstates;
                                                e(i)+r(i)/nt*ott;
                                                r(i)+(-ot(i));
                                                o(i) + ot(i);
                                                d(i)+ (o(i)-e(i));
                                        end;
                                    nt+(-ott);
                                    output;
                        end;
                          end;
     data ddd;
             set dd end=last;
             array e(*) e1-e&nstates;
             array o(*) o1-o&nstates; if last;
             df=&nstates-1;
             do &state=1 to &nstates;
                     expected=e(&state); observed=o(&state);
                            ratio=observed/expected;
                     diff=observed-expected;
                     output;
                     end;
     data cov;
             set ddd;
             keep v1-v&nstat2;
             %let slist=;
             %do i=1 %to &nstates;
                     data _null_ ;
                            call symput('s', put(&i,&format));
                     run;
                     %let slist= &slist &s ;
                     %end;
     data exp ;
             set ddd;
             keep e1-e&nstates;
     data obs;
             set ddd;
             keep o1-o&nstates;

     /* Use IML to calculate test statistic and print results */

     proc iml;
             use cov;
             read into covmat;
             cov=shape(covmat,&nstates);
             statlist={&slist};
             tranlist=statlist';
             use exp;
             read into expmat;
             print 'Covariance Matrix';
             print cov[r=tranlist c=statlist format=10.4];
             v=diag(cov);
             use obs;
             read into obsmat;
             rmat=obsmat#expmat##(-1);
             r=rmat';
          difmat=obsmat-expmat;
          d=difmat';
            obs=obsmat'; exp=expmat';
            z=difmat*inv(v##(.5));
            p=(1-probnorm(abs(z)))'; p=2*p;
            state =state  =obs||exp||r||d||p;
            top={'Observed' 'Expected' 'O/E' 'O-E' 'P-Value'};
            print 'Summary of Results for Each State';
            print state[r=tranlist c=top format=12.4];
            cov=cov[1:&nml,1:&nml];
            expmat =expmat[1,1:&nml];
            obsmat=obsmat[1,1:&nml];
            chisq=(expmat-obsmat)*inv(cov)*(expmat-obsmat)';
            print 'Test of Homogeneity of States';
            p=1-probchi(chisq,&nml);
            df=&nml;
            print chisq [format=11.4] df [format=5.0] p [format=8.4] ;
     %mend mantbyar;
```

Chapter 4   Proportional Hazards Regression

1. The Cox (Proportional Hazards) Regression Method

1.1 The Basic Model

In Chapter 3, "Nonparametric Comparison of Survival Distributions," you learned how to compare groups with respect to survival. The methods presented were valid without regard to any assumptions concerning the survival distributions of the groups. In this chapter, you learn how to analyze the effect of a numeric variable on survival. The method, known as Cox regression, or proportional hazards regression, was introduced by Cox (1972). It is based on a model known as the Cox model, or proportional hazards model. This model assumes that additive changes in the value of a numeric variable cause corresponding multiplicative changes in the hazard function. The SAS procedure PHREG, which implements this method, is discussed in this chapter.

Consider a population in which a variable, x, is observed in addition to the survival time and censoring variables. Such a variable is called a *covariate*. For now, only one such covariate is considered. The extension to more than one follows. Let $h(t, x)$ be the hazard function that gives the hazard at time t for an individual having a value of x for the covariate. Then, the proportional hazards model assumes the following for some parameter, β:

$$h(t, x) = h_0(t)\exp(\beta x) \tag{1}$$

The function, $h_0(t)$ is called the *underlying hazard function*. Note that it is independent of x. In fact, it is the hazard function of a patient for whom $x = 0$. This assumption implies that a unit increase in x multiplies the hazard by the same value for all values of t, namely $\exp(\beta)$. Of course, the key to analysis of survival with this model is to estimate β and make inferences about its value. For example, if the hypothesis $\beta = 0$ is rejected, then it can be inferred that the variable x influences the hazard, and hence, the survival function. If $\beta > 0$, then the hazard increases (and survival worsens) as x increases. Similarly, if $\beta < 0$, then the hazard decreases (and survival improves) as x increases. The estimated value of β leads to an estimate of $\exp(\beta)$, which is the value of the ratio $h(t, x + 1)/h(t, x)$ for all values of t and x. That ratio is called the *hazard ratio*. Sometimes this ratio is called the *risk ratio* and is abbreviated RR.

Although this model is often employed for continuous covariates, it is also appropriate for a dichotomous covariate, such as treatment group. If treatment group is coded as 0 or 1, then $\exp(\beta)$ is the ratio of the hazard for group 1 to the hazard for group 0. That ratio is assumed to be constant for all time. Thus, the method of this chapter provides an alternative to the log rank test and the other linear rank tests of Chapter 3.

1.2 The Proportional Hazards Assumption

It should be noted that the proportional hazards assumption that underlies this model is fairly strong and may not always be reasonable. Consider a covariate x, which equals 1 for a surgical intervention and 0 for a non-surgical intervention. Suppose that the surgical intervention has high early risk, but once a patient has survived the surgery and its effects, prospects for long term survival are excellent. On the other hand, the non-surgical intervention does not have high early risk, but it does not have very good long term survival either. In this case, the risk ratio might be high initially, but it decreases as time increases. For another example, consider the covariate of age at diagnosis. It might be the case that hazard increases considerably as age increases from 60 to 70 years old, but very little or not at all as age increases from 15 to 25 years old. The proportional hazards assumption implies that $h(t, 70)/h(t, 60) = h(t, 25)/h(t, 15)$ for all values of t. In both of these examples the proportional hazards assumption would not be valid, and the method of this chapter would be inappropriate. Ways to study the validity of the proportional hazards assumption are considered later in this chapter.

2. Multiple Covariates

Now suppose that, for each patient, you observe P covariates, which you label $x_1, x_2, \ldots, x_P$. Then, for each patient, there is a corresponding column vector $\mathbf{x} = (x_1, x_2, \ldots, x_P)'$ of covariates. Let $h(t, \mathbf{x})$ be the hazard function at t for a patient whose covariates have values given by the components of $\mathbf{x}$. To extend the proportional hazards model to multiple covariates, it is assumed that, for some vector of parameters $\beta = (\beta_1, \beta_2, \ldots, \beta_P)'$

$$h(t, \mathbf{x}) = h_0(t)\exp(\beta'\mathbf{x}) \tag{2}$$

Since $\beta'\mathbf{x} = \beta_1 x_1 + \beta_2 x_2 + \ldots + \beta_P x_P$, this means that the proportional hazards assumption holds for each of the individual covariates with the others held constant. This model allows for the estimation of the effect of each covariate in the presence of the others. As in the univariate case, the focus of the analyses is the estimation of the parameters, $\beta_1, \beta_2, \ldots, \beta_P$. The risk ratio for x_j is given by $\exp(\beta_j)$, and the risk ratio for any set of the covariates is the product of their risk ratios.

3. Defining Covariates

3.1 Interactions

Interactions among the covariates, that is, the tendency of the effect of one covariate on survival to vary according to the value of another covariate, can be studied by defining new covariates as products of the original covariates. For example, suppose that x_1 is a covariate that takes on the value of 0 or 1 depending upon the treatment group, and that x_2 is a patient's weight. If you wish to include the interaction of weight and treatment in the model, you can introduce a new covariate, x_3, that is defined as $x_1 x_2$. Now suppose that PROC PHREG indicates that β_3 is positive. What does that mean? To answer this question, write equation 2 as

$$h(t, x_1, x_2, x_3) = h_0(t)\exp[\beta_1 x_1 + (\beta_2 + \beta_3 x_1)x_2] \tag{3}$$

When $x_1 = 0$, each additional unit of x_2 multiplies the hazard at any time by $\exp(\beta_2)$. But when $x_1 = 1$, each additional unit of x_2 multiplies the hazard at any time by $\exp(\beta_2 + \beta_3)$. Thus, if β_3 is positive, the effect of weight is greater in group 1 than in group 0. By writing the exponent in equation 3 as $\beta_2 x_2 + (\beta_1 + \beta_3 x_2)x_1$, you can see another interpretation. The group effect is greater among heavier patients.

3.2 Categorical Variables with More than Two Values

You may sometimes have a grouping variable that takes on more than two values. For example, you might be studying a type of cancer with four main histologies. For convenience, call them A, B, C, and D. This variable can be studied by the methods above by converting histology into three covariates as follows:

x_1 which is 1 for histology A, 0 otherwise.

x_2 which is 1 for histology B, 0 otherwise.

x_3 which is 1 for histology C, 0 otherwise.

Do not define a fourth covariate, x_4, for histology D. If you do so, the values of the four covariates will sum to 1 for every patient, creating a numerical problem.

If β_1 is the coefficient of x_1 in the model of expression 2, then $\exp(\beta_1)$ is the ratio of the hazard for those with histology A to the hazard for those with histology D. Similar statements can be made for the coefficients of x_2 and x_3. For i and j chosen from 1, 2, and 3, $\exp(\beta_i - \beta_j)$ is the ratio of the hazard for the histology represented by x_i to the hazard of the histology represented by x_j.

3.3 Scaling the Covariates

It is tempting not to be concerned about the scale in which covariates are measured. After all, the question of whether a patient's weight affects survival should, with any reasonable statistical method, be answered the same whether weight is measured in kilograms, pounds, grams, or tons. In fact, that is the case for proportional hazards regression. However, the scale used can make large differences in the estimate of the hazard ratio and lead to results that are easily misinterpreted.

To make the discussion specific, suppose that a covariate is measured in millimeters and that PROC PHREG produces an estimate of 0.049 for its beta coefficient and, thus, an estimate of $\exp(0.049) = 1.05$ for its risk ratio. That means that a millimeter increase in the covariate is estimated to increase the hazard by 5%. An increase of 10 millimeters, or 1 centimeter, would then multiply the hazard by $1.05^{10} = 1.63$. If the analysis were done with the covariate measured in centimeters, the estimate of the beta coefficient would be $10 \times 0.049 = 0.49$, and the estimated risk ratio would be 1.63. The lesson here is that it is important to report the unit of measurement along with the hazard ratio for a continuous variable.

A more extreme situation can result from dealing with covariates based on dates, such as a patient's age at diagnosis. Suppose age is simply defined in a SAS DATA step as date of diagnosis minus date of birth. This will produce, of course, the patient's age in days. If PROC PHREG produced an estimated risk ratio of 1.0001, you might be inclined to think that the effect of age is minimal. However, this would be equivalent to a risk ratio of 1.44 ($= 1.0001^{3650}$) for a decade of age. Thus a 50 year old would have 44% greater hazard than a 40 year old.

4. Survival Probabilities

Until now the discussion has dealt with the hazard function. When analyzing survival data, however, you are probably more concerned with survival probabilities and how they are affected by the values of the covariates under study. Recalling equation 7 of Chapter 1, if we let $S(t, \mathbf{x})$ represent the value of the survival function at time t for a patient with covariate vector $\mathbf{x}$, the proportional hazards model implies that

$$S(t, \mathbf{x}) = \exp[-\int_0^t h_0(u) e^{\beta'x} du] \tag{4}$$

But the right hand side can be written as

$$\{\exp[-H_0(t)]\}^{\exp(\beta'\mathbf{x})} \tag{5}$$

where $H_0(t)$ is the integral $\int_0^t h_0(u) du$. That integral is called the *baseline cumulative hazard*.

Once we have estimates for the beta's, survival probabilities can be estimated if we can estimate this baseline cumulative hazard. In fact, as will be discussed later in this chapter, PROC PHREG can do this as well.

Now suppose that two patients have covariate vectors that differ by 1 in covariate x_j but not in any other covariate. Then, their exponents $\exp(\beta'\mathbf{x})$ in equation 5 differ by the factor $\exp(\beta_j)$. But that is what was previously called the risk ratio for covariate x_j. Thus a risk ratio of r affects survival probabilities by raising them to the rth power. For example, if a risk ratio for a group with a covariate value of 1 relative to the group having the covariate value of 0 is 2.0, then, for any time, t, the survival probability for group 1 at t is the square of the corresponding survival probability for group 0. At a time for which that probability is 0.60 in group 0, that probability will be 0.36 in group 1.

5. Using PROC PHREG

5.1 Basic Usage

In order to use PROC PHREG, you should have, for each patient, a time variable and a censoring (or event) variable to indicate survival status. In addition, you will have values for one or more covariates that you wish to analyze for possible effect on survival. To invoke the procedure, you need the procedure statement, followed by a MODEL statement giving the time and (optionally) censoring variable, and the covariates to be used in the analysis. The basic syntax looks like this:

```
proc phreg;
     model timevar*censvar(censval(s)) = covariate(s);
```

Here, *timevar* is the time variable and *censvar* is the censoring variable. If no observations are censored, then *censvar* is not needed. *censval(s)* are the values of *censvar* that indicate that a time is censored. *covariate(s)* is the list of variables to be considered as the covariates of the regression. The MODEL statement can also include an option to specify how ties in the time variable are handled. The default is to use a method due to Breslow (1974). This will generally be satisfactory. PROC PHREG uses only those observations for which all of these variables are nonmissing. You might, therefore, be cautious about including covariates for which many patients have missing values.

Since Release 6.10, SAS has permitted an alternative version of the MODEL statement. In this version, *timevar* is replaced by a pair of time variables of the form *(t1, t2)*. These variables are the left and right endpoints of the time interval during which the patient was at risk of experiencing the event being studied. For the situations we have been dealing with, the left endpoint is always 0 and the right endpoint is always the same time variable we have already been using. This form of the MODEL statement does permit you to deal with some more complex situations, however. For example, you can deal with events that can occur multiple times to each patient, such as tumor recurrence or the onset of a migraine headache. A patient for whom the event being studied occurred twice, say at times 6 and 11 before censoring at time 15, would have three observations in the data set. The associated time variables would have the values 0 and 6 for the first observation, 6 and 11 for the second, and 11 and 15 for the third. The censoring variable would have a value indicating an uncensored observation for the first two observations and a value used for a censored observation for the third.

Estimation of the beta's is accomplished by maximizing what is known as the partial likelihood that is defined in terms of the survival data and the patients' covariate values. The critical feature of this method is that it does not require any knowledge or assumptions concerning the underlying hazard function, $h_0(t)$. Further details of the principles underlying likelihood-based estimation and hypothesis testing are provided at the end of this chapter.

The output includes estimates of the beta coefficients and the associated risk ratios. Estimates of the standard errors of the coefficients are also given. The beta coefficient estimates are each approximately normally distributed, with mean zero, under the null hypothesis that the covariate has no effect on survival. Thus, if $\hat{\beta}$ is the estimate of β and s is its estimated standard error, $(\hat{\beta}/s)^2$ has, approximately, a χ^2 distribution with 1 degree of freedom under the null hypothesis. This statistic, and its associated *p*-value, are also given. In addition, three test statistics for the hypothesis that all the parameters are 0 are reported.

5.2 An Example

Consider the following analysis of a cohort of melanoma patients. The investigator had survival data on these patients as well as the year, from 1988 to 1993, in which they were diagnosed and the thickness, in millimeters, of the tumor. He was interested in the effect of both of these variables on survival. The following statements were used:

```
proc phreg;
        model time*censor(0)= year thicknes;
```

The output is given as Output 4.1.

Output 4.1

```
                        The SAS System

                     The PHREG Procedure

Data Set: WORK.DATA1
Dependent Variable: TIME
Censoring Variable: CENSOR        ❶
Censoring Value(s): 0
Ties Handling: BRESLOW

                    Summary of the Number of
                    Event and Censored Values

                                            Percent
            Total       Event    Censored   Censored

            749          73        676       90.25          ❷


          Testing Global Null Hypothesis: BETA=0    ❸

            Without     With
Criterion Covariates Covariates Model Chi-Square

-2 LOG L      862.825    833.211    29.614 with 2 DF (p=0.0001)
Score           .          .        44.217 with 2 DF (p=0.0001)
Wald            .          .        41.229 with 2 DF (p=0.0001)
```

```
        Analysis of Maximum Likelihood Estimates        ❹

                Parameter    Standard     Wald        Pr >
Variable   DF    Estimate      Error   Chi-Square  Chi-Square

THICKNES   1     0.200125     0.03330   36.11637     0.0001
YEAR       1    -0.234093     0.11264    4.31928     0.0377

    Analysis of
Maximum Likelihood      ❺
    Estimates


              Risk
Variable     Ratio

THICKNES     1.222
YEAR         0.791
```

The output presents the following:

❶ information about the data set used, the time and censoring variables, and the method of handling ties.

❷ the number of observations and the number censored.

❸ three tests of the null hypothesis that all of the covariates are zero. In this case they all are highly significant, indicating that at least one of the covariates affects the hazard, hence, survival.

❹ estimates of each of the beta coefficients and standard errors of the estimates. The Wald χ^2 is the square of the ratio of the estimated coefficient to its standard error. Each p-value, based on a χ^2 distribution with 1 degree of freedom is also given. As with other SAS procedure output, a p-value of 0.0001 is given whenever the actual p-value is less than or equal to that value. In fact, the p-value for a χ^2 statistic with 1 degree of freedom that exceeds 36 is much smaller than that. The positive sign of the estimated parameters associated with tumor thickness and its p-value indicates that hazard is increased, hence survival probabilities diminished, for thicker tumors. Similarly, the negative sign for the estimated parameter associated with the year of diagnosis indicates that the hazard is decreased, hence survival probabilities increased, for the melanomas diagnosed in the later years.

❺ the hazard ratios, which are just the antilog of the parameters. They indicate that, when adjusting for the year diagnosed, each millimeter of increased tumor thickness increases the hazard by 22%. Also, adjusting for the tumor thickness, the hazard for tumors diagnosed in each year is 79% of the hazard for the previous year.

5.3 Statements Used with PROC PHREG

PROC PHREG has a rich collection of additional features that you can use. Only those that are most useful are discussed here. As with many other SAS procedures, a statement of the form

```
by varname;
```

causes separate analyses to be done for each value of *varname*, and a statement of the form

```
where expression;
```

causes the analyses to be on only those patients for whom *expression* is true. A statement of the form

```
strata varname(s);
```

causes a stratified analysis to be done. A stratified analysis allows you to adjust for certain variables that are not thought to have the proportional hazards property. Strata are formed for each combination of the values of *varname(s)*. Numeric variables can be followed by lists, such as (0 TO 100 BY 10) or (0 TO 5, 5.1 TO 10, 10.1 TO 20), to create stratum levels. The list of statification variables can be followed by the MISSING option to cause missing values for the stratification variables to be treated as valid variable values. Without this specification, patients for whom any of the stratification variables have a missing value are excluded from the analysis. The way that PROC PHREG performs a stratified analysis is discussed at the end of this chapter.

There are also statements that can be used to produce estimates of survival functions over time for specified values of the covariates. These are discussed later in this chapter.

5.4 Options Used with the Procedure Statement and MODEL Statement

5.4.1 Options that Produce Additional Output

Specifying the SIMPLE option in the PROC PHREG statement causes simple descriptive statistics for each variable in the right side of the model statement to be printed. Several important options can be specified in the MODEL statement. They must follow a slash (/) that follows the independent variables. RISKLIMITS, or RL, causes the output to include $(100 - \alpha)100\%$ confidence intervals for the risk ratios. The default value for α is 0.05. This can be altered by ALPHA = *value*.

5.4.2 Options that Direct Model Building

There are several options, called *model-building options*, that control which of a set of covariates that you supply actually get used in the model. These options are used when you are looking for a set of covariates that can distinquish patients with respect to patients' anticipated survival prospects. Using these options is tricky and somewhat controversial among statisticians. Some argue that such methods should not be used at all. After a description of these methods and an example of their use is given, this chapter discusses some problems and things you should think about when using these methods.

By using the option SELECTION = FORWARD, you cause the covariates that are to be included in the model to be chosen one at a time. The procedure starts by performing univariate proportional hazards regressions with each independent variable in the MODEL statement. The variable with the largest score χ^2 is entered into the model. The procedure then performs the two variable proportional hazards regressions by using each of the remaining covariates with the one already chosen. The covariate with the largest score χ^2 in the model containing the first one entered is then added to the model. The process continues in this fashion until none of the remaining covariates have score χ^2 values large enough to be included. The default is for the process to stop when none of the remaining covariates is significant at the 0.05 level. Other values can be chosen by including the option SLENTRY (or SLE) = *value*. If you wish to wish to limit the model to *n* covariates, you can use the option STOP = *n*. If you wish to force *m* particular covariates to be included in the model, you can list them first in the MODEL statement and use the option START = *m*.

There are other model building options that can be used to build models in different ways. Using SELECTION = STEPWISE causes the procedure to go through a process similar to the one previously described for SELECTION = FORWARD. The difference is that SELECTION = STEPWISE allows covariates previously entered to be removed from the model if they are no longer significant using the Wald χ^2 statistic. The default threshold for significance is 0.05. This can be altered by using the option SLSTAY = *value* where *value* is the desired significance threshold. Again the process stops when all of the covariates not in the model have score χ^2 *p*-values exceeding the SLE value. The process also stops if a covariate is entered into the model and then removed in the same step. If the process did not stop under this condition, you could have that covariate both entered and removed indefinitely.

The option SELECTION = BACKWARD causes the procedure to begin by estimating the coeficients for all of the covariates in the MODEL statement. The covariate that has the smallest value for the 1 degree of freedom Wald χ^2 statistic is then removed from the model if the *p*-value for that covariate is larger than the SLSTAY value specified. The default is 0.05. The process stops when all of the covariates still in the model have Wald χ^2 *p*-values smaller than the SLSTAY value.

Another way to specify the models created is to use the options SELECTION = SCORE and BEST = *n*. These will cause the best *n* models of each size to be found and printed. Best, in this case, means having the highest score statistic. That statistic is one of the three described earlier that provide a measure of the collective significance of the covariates in the model. For example, if ten covariates are specified in the MODEL statement and the options SELECTION = SCORE and BEST = 5 are used, then the procedure prints out the five best one-covariate models, the five best two-covariate models, and so on, until it gets to the five best nine-covariate models. Of course, there is only one ten-covariate model. It will be printed out as well. If the BEST = n option is omitted and there are ten or fewer covariates in the MODEL statement, then the procedure will print all models with each number of covariates. If you think that can be a lot of models, you are right. With ten covariates, this will result in $2^{10} - 1 = 1023$ models being printed. If there are more than ten covariates in the MODEL statement, then the number of models of each size printed will not exceed the number of covariates.

5.5 A Model Building Example

For an example of the use of PROC PHREG for creating a proportional hazards model for survival based on a set of survival data and covariate values, another melanoma data set is considered. The data are based on 968 patients who had their melanomas surgically removed. Disease-free survival (DFS) time is defined as the time, in months, until either death or tumor relapse. Several covariates are recorded and analyzed for association with DFS. Location is coded as 1, 2, 3, or 4. Sex was coded as 0 for females and 1 for males. Breslow score is a measure of the tumor's thickness, and Clark score is a measure of how far it has spread. The presence or absence of ulcers is coded as 1 or 0, respectively. Three dichotomous location covariates are defined as described in section 3.2 of this chapter. LOC1 equals 1 if the location is 1, 0 otherwise. LOC2 and LOC3 are defined similarly.

A forward selection method is used with the default significance threshold of 0.05. Ninety-five percent confidence intervals are requested with the RL option. The DETAILS option causes details of the selection process to be printed.

The following SAS statements produce Output 4.2:

```
proc phreg;
    model dfstime*dfscens(0) = loc1-loc3 sex clark breslow ulcer/
    selection = forward rl details;
    title1 'Porportional Hazards Regression Analysis';
    title2 'Of Melanoma Data';
```

Output 4.2

```
                    Proportional Hazards Regression Analysis
                              Of Melanoma Data

                           The PHREG Procedure

Data Set: WORK.DATA
Dependent Variable: DFSTIME
Censoring Variable: DFSCENS
Censoring Value(s): 0
Ties Handling: BRESLOW


                          Summary of the Number of
                          Event and Censored Values


                                                   Percent
               Total        Event    Censored     Censored

                968          201        767         79.24

               Analysis of Variables Not in the Model


                                 Score           Pr >
               Variable      Chi-Square      Chi-Square

               LOC1             1.0273          0.3108
               LOC2             0.0283          0.8663
    ❶          LOC3             3.0090          0.0828
               SEX              1.8951          0.1686
               CLARK           37.1010          0.0001
               BRESLOW         73.9724          0.0001
               ULCER           24.9179          0.0001


    ❷    Residual Chi-square = 80.7527   with 7 DF (p=0.0001)


Step  1: Variable BRESLOW is entered.  The model contains the
          following explanatory variables.


    ❸       BRESLOW
               Testing Global Null Hypothesis: BETA=0


               Without      With
Criterion    Covariates  Covariates  Model Chi-Square


-2 LOG L      2274.798    2219.676     55.122 with 1 DF (p=0.0001)
Score            .            .        73.972 with 1 DF (p=0.0001)    ❹
Wald             .            .        72.961 with 1 DF (p=0.0001)
```

```
              Analysis of Maximum Likelihood Estimates

                    Parameter    Standard     Wald        Pr >
 Variable   DF       Estimate      Error    Chi-Square  Chi-Square

 BRESLOW     1       0.338195     0.03959    72.96063     0.0001   ❺


   Analysis of Maximum Likelihood Estimates

              Conditional Risk Ratio and
                95% Confidence Limits

                  Risk
 Variable         Ratio        Lower        Upper

 BRESLOW          1.402        1.298        1.516   ❺

           Analysis of Variables Not in the Model

                             Score          Pr >
                Variable   Chi-Square     Chi-Square

                LOC1          2.3063        0.1289
                LOC2          0.2266        0.6341
      ❻        LOC3          2.0602        0.1512
                SEX           0.3358        0.5623
                CLARK         9.5331        0.0020
                ULCER         2.5655        0.1092

   ❼  Residual Chi-square = 14.6913   with 6 DF (p=0.0228)


Step  2: Variable CLARK is entered.  The model contains the
         following explanatory variables.

         CLARK      BRESLOW

           Testing Global Null Hypothesis: BETA=0

           Without    With
Criterion Covariates Covariates Model Chi-Square

-2 LOG L   2274.798   2209.735   65.063 with 2 DF (p=0.0001)
Score         .          .       75.800 with 2 DF (p=0.0001)  ❽
Wald          .          .       69.789 with 2 DF (p=0.0001)
```

```
         Analysis of Maximum Likelihood Estimates    ❾

                Parameter    Standard     Wald       Pr >
Variable  DF    Estimate      Error    Chi-Square  Chi-Square

CLARK     1     0.369258     0.12024    9.43189     0.0021
BRESLOW   1     0.264874     0.04847   29.85701     0.0001


   Analysis of Maximum Likelihood Estimates

           Conditional Risk Ratio and
              95% Confidence Limits

             Risk
Variable     Ratio      Lower        Upper

CLARK        1.447      1.143        1.831      ❾
BRESLOW      1.303      1.185        1.433

         Analysis of Variables Not in the Model

                         Score        Pr >
              Variable  Chi-Square  Chi-Square

              LOC1       1.1964      0.2740
              LOC2       0.0763      0.7824
    ❿         LOC3       1.6817      0.1947
              SEX        0.0580      0.8097
              ULCER      2.0892      0.1483

❶❶      Residual Chi-square = 5.3010  with 5 DF (p=0.3803)

NOTE: No (additional) variables met the 0.05 level for entry
      into the model.

❶❷      Summary of Forward Selection Procedure

           Variable   Number     Score       Pr >
     Step   Entered     In     Chi-Square  Chi-Square

       1   BRESLOW      1       73.9724     0.0001   ❾
       2   CLARK        2        9.5331     0.0020
```

Note the following features of the output:

❶ The seven univariate proportional hazards regression models are calculated.

❷ The highly significant residual χ^2 indicates that the model containing the seven covariates is superior to the model with none of them.

❸ Breslow, the most highly significant of the seven covariates, is entered into the model.

❹ Three tests of the significance of the model containing Breslow are reported. All are highly significant.

❺ The estimated beta coefficient for Breslow in the one-covariate model, its standard error, and its significance level are given. An estimate of the relative risk associated with a Breslow increase of one unit is given as well as a 95% confidence interval for that relative risk.

❻ Score χ^2 statistics, along with their *p*-values for the six two-covariate proportional hazards models using Breslow and each of the remaining covariates, are computed. The highest χ^2 value is for the model in which Clark is added.

❼ The residual χ^2 is significant, indicating that at least one of the remaining variables is relevant in determining survival probabilities.

❽ Clark is added to the model. The three statistics for the two-covariate model are calculated. All are significant.

❾ Beta coefficient estimates, their standard errors, and their significance level for each of the two covariates now in the model are reported. Estimates of the risk ratios and 95% confidence intervals for each of the covariates are also given.

❿ The five three-covariate proportional hazards regressions using Breslow, Clark, and each of the remaining five covariates are calculated. None meet the significance threshold of 0.05.

⓫ residual χ^2 is not significant, indicating no evidence that the remaining covariates influence survival.

⓬ The model building process ends. A summary of the covariate selection process is given.

It is interesting to note that the presence of ulcers was significant when considered in isolation, but does not appear in the final model. Apparently it is highly correlated with Breslow. Those patients with ulcers tend to have high Breslow scores. Thus, with Breslow in the model, the presence of ulcers is no longer significant.

6. Model Building Considerations

6.1 Correlated Covariates

Other SAS procedures, LOGISTIC and REG, have model building options similar to those described above. The remarks that follow apply to these procedures as well. First of all, you need to be aware that the different methods can, and often do, produce different final models. Each has some logical basis, and it would be difficult to say that one is better than the others. Also you need to realize that a covariate that is left out of, or omitted from, the model may, on its own, be highly significant. That can happen if that covariate happens to be highly correlated with a covariate (or a linear combination of covariates) that are currently in the model. Suppose, for example, that x_1 and x_2 have score χ^2's in univariate proportional hazard regressions of 5.62 and 5.64 respectively. Then, in a stepwise or forward selection, x_2 will be entered into the model. Now if x_1 and x_2 are highly correlated, then x_1 may not be significant in the model containing x_2. Thus x_1 will not appear in the model. If another sample were similarly analyzed, x_1 might, simply by chance, have a larger χ^2 than x_2. Thus, it would be entered into the model and x_2 might be left out.

6.2 The "Multiple Testing" Problem

Another thing you need to realize is that the p-values reported for each covariate in a final model in which the covariates are a subset of a larger set are seriously biased. With a large number of covariates in the model, the probability that at least one will be considered "significant" and entered into the model is much higher than the stated or default SLENTRY value. For example, if a MODEL statement lists 25 independent covariates that are not related to survival at all and SLENTRY = 0.05, then there is a probability of 0.72 that at least one will be "significant" and entered into the model with a p-value less than 0.05, and a probability of 0.36 that at least two will. For this reason, you should avoid thoughtlessly putting a large number a covariates into a MODEL statement. Use only covariates that make sense clinically or biologically. Even so, models created in one of the ways described above need to be confirmed on additional data sets. If you have a sample size that is large enough, you might want to divide it into parts. Use one part to build a model and the other to test it.

6.3 Pre-Screening Covariates

As noted in Section 5.1, a patient will be excluded from the analysis if any of the covariates in the MODEL statement have missing values. Unfortunately, missing values are very common when dealing with medical data. Tests that are supposed to generate values of the covariates are sometimes not done. Sometimes clinical problems prevent their being done. Sometimes tests are done, but the results are technically inadequate or equivocal. With a large number of covariates, even if each is nonmissing for 90% to 95% of the patients, you might have data on all of the covariates for less than half of the patients in the sample. One way to lessen this problem is to pre-screen the covariates with univariate proportional hazard regressions. You would then perform a second proportional hazards regression using only those covariates passing through the first screen with p-values less than some threshold value, say 0.05 or 0.10. In this way, missing values for covariates that are apparently not associated with survival and are unlikely to wind up in the final model will not cause a patient to be excluded.

6.4 Grouping Covariates

Sometimes there are great differences in the cost of acquiring values for covariates. The term "cost" is used here in a broad sense to include such factors as risk to the patient, morbidity, inconvenience, and so on. It is only reasonable to consider these factors in determining a model for hazard. A covariate might be highly associated with prognosis and thus provide a useful guide to therapy. However, its determination might cause considerable morbidity or be very expensive. We would prefer to avoid obtaining it if another covariate, or group of covariates, can provide the same information. One way to accomplish this is to group the covariates according to the costs associated with their determination. Then, do a series of proportional hazards regressions using those of less cost in the earlier steps. In each step, add the covariates in the next group to those added to the model in the previous steps.

For purposes of illustration, suppose that you have three such groups, which you label A, B, and C, with group A being the least costly to acquire and group C being the most costly. First run PROC PHREG with some model building options on the covariates in group A only. Presumably, n of them will be in the final model. Then, re-run PROC PHREG with these n covariates listed first in the MODEL statement, followed by those in group B using the option START = n. This will cause the n covariates from the first step to be included as well as the m group B covariates that are significant in the model containing these covariates. Now run PROC PHREG once again listing the $m + n$ covariates from this second model first, followed by the covariates in group C. Use the option START = r where $r = n+m$. This procedure ensures that a covariate is in the final model only if it has an influence on the hazard, hence survival, that is not accounted for by covariates that are less costly to acquire.

6.5 Using Cutpoints on a Continuous Covariate

When dealing with a continuous covariate, you have two approaches that you can use. One is to use the actual value that is observed in a Cox regression as described above. The other is to convert it to a dichotomous covariate, or perhaps an ordinal covariate, by using cutpoints. For example, instead of using the age of a woman with breast cancer, you can create a dichotomous covariate to use. This covariate would take on the value 0 if the woman is 60 years old or less, and 1 if the woman is over 60 years old. This covariate could be used in a proportional hazards regression or as the grouping variable in one of the linear rank tests discussed in Chapter 3. Arguments can be made for and against both approaches. Here are two arguments against the use of cutpoints:

- By converting from a continuous variable to a dichotomous variable, you are throwing out potentially useful information. After all, ages of 47, 62, or 85 are more informative than "less than 60" or "greater than 60". It doesn't make sense to consider a 59 year old and a 61 year old to be different but a 62 year old and an 85 year old to be the same.

- The choice of a cutpoint or cutpoints is arbitrary. If dichotomizing age, for example, where do you draw the line? Using a cutpoint of 50 might lead to a statistically significant beta coefficient, while a cutpoint of 60 might not. You might simply use the median value of the covariate. Many analysts will try a variety of cutpoints and use the one with the largest χ^2 statistic. If you do that, you need to understand that the resultant p-value is subject to the multiple testing effect discussed in section 6.2. A recent report (Altman et al. 1994) and a letter commenting on it (Cantor and Shuster, 1994) discuss this issue in greater detail.

Here are two arguments for the use of cutpoints:

- Although it might be reasonable to assume that the effect of a covariate's value on the hazard function is monotonic, it might not be reasonable to assume that it is exponential, as required by the proportional hazards model. The hazard ratio for an 80 year old versus a 70 year old might differ from the corresponding ratio for a 50 year old versus a 40 year old. Dichotomizing age avoids this problem.

- The results for a dichotomous variable are easier to interpret to others, particularly those not statistically sophisticated. It is easier for such a person to understand (or at least to think he understands) that older patients have a 40% greater risk (i.e. a risk ratio of 1.40) than that each year increases the risk by 3% (i.e., a risk ratio of 1.03 per year). In fact, if a continuous covariate is dichotomized, then the log rank test or one of the other linear rank tests can be used. Then, the results can be interpreted in terms of the observed versus expected number of deaths in each group. This is a convenient way to visualize the magnitude of the effect of a dichotomous variable.

There is no single simple answer to the question of whether it is better to use the actual value of a continuous covariate or to dichotomize it with a cutpoint. You need to consider the way that you expect the covariate to affect survival, as well as the anticipated audience for your analyses, and decide accordingly.

7. Time Dependent Covariates

The method of proportional hazards regression and PROC PHREG can be used in a manner that has not yet been discussed. You may want to consider the effect on survival of a covariate that is not constant over time. Such a covariate is called a *time dependent covariate*. Some examples might be a patient's weight, diastolic blood pressure, or level of certain serum markers. A dichotomous variable might also vary with time. Consider patients who are candidates for an organ transplant. They are followed from the time at which that determination is made, but it might be some time before the transplant can be accomplished. Some will die before receiving a transplant. Others may die post-transplant. To study the effect of transplantation on survival, you can consider "transplantation state" as a covariate. If the patient is transplanted at time t_0, then that covariate can be assigned a value of 0 for $t < t_0$ and 1 for $t \geq t_0$. In Chapter 3, you saw how the Mantel-Byar method could be used to analyze such data. The following technique offers an alternative approach.

Notation of the form $x(t)$ is used for a covariate that may vary over time. The column vector $(x_1(t), x_2(t), \ldots, x_p(t))'$ is denoted $\mathbf{x}(t)$. The proportional hazards regression model can then be written

$$h[t, \mathbf{x}(t)] = h_0(t)\exp[\boldsymbol{\beta}'\mathbf{x}(t)] \qquad (6)$$

where $\boldsymbol{\beta}$ is, as before, a column vector of regression coefficients.

If $x(t)$ is a time dependent covariate that you wish to consider in a proportional hazards regression, you need to provide information on the value of x for all values of t. This is done through programming statements that follow the MODEL statement. These statements can use many of the statements, and all of the functions, that can be used in the DATA step. As an example, suppose you are following patients who are candidates for an organ transplant. That data might contain the variables TIME, for the patients' time on study, and CENSOR, to indicate whether the patient was alive (0) or dead (1). In addition you might have a variable, TRANTIME, that represents the time at which the patient was transplanted. If the patient never received a transplant, this variable would have a missing value. The following SAS statements could be used to do a proportional hazards regression analysis with "transplant state," which is denoted by TRANS as a time dependent covariate:

```
proc phreg;
    model time*censor(0) = trans;
    trans = 0;
    if time ge trantime and trantime ne . then trans = 1;
run;
```

A positive value for the coefficient of TRANS would indicate that, as the value of TRANS increased (i.e., went from 0 to 1), the hazard was increased and thus survival was diminished. In other words, a positive value for this coefficient indicates that transplantation is deleterious. Similarly, a negative value for the coefficient of trans would indicate that transplantation was helpful.

Continuous time dependent covariates cause greater trouble. Generally, you could not monitor a patient continuously for values of such a covariate. Even if you could, how would you translate the values for that function into programming statements? Instead, what is usually done is to record values of the covariate at certain times, say $t_1, t_2, \ldots, t_k$ where $t_1 = 0$. Suppose those corresponding values are $a_1, a_2, \ldots, a_k$. Then, the programming statements to assign, for any time, the most recently recorded value might look like this (for $k=10$):

```
array t{10};
array a{10};
x = a1;
do i = 1 to 10;
    if t{i} ne . and time ge t{i} then x = a{i};
    end;
run;
```

By using time dependent covariates, you can also create more complex models in situations where the proportional hazards property does not hold. To reprise an example mentioned in section 1.2 of this chapter, let $x_1 = 1$ if a patient was treated surgically and 0 otherwise. Suppose you believe that the hazard ratio is different after $t = 90$ days from the hazard ratio prior to that time. You might use the following statements to analyze the survival data:

```
proc phreg;
    model t*cens(0)= x1 x2;
    if t < 90 then x2 = 0;
    else x2 = x1;
```

Now suppose β_1 and β_2 are the regression coeficients for x_1 and x_2 respectively. Then the hazard function can be written $h(t, x_1, x_2) = h_0(t)\exp[\beta_1 x_1 + \beta_2 x_2(t)]$. This means that the x_1 (surgery) effect is β_1 prior to $t = 90$ and $\beta_1 + \beta_2$ thereafter. If surgery is associated with increased hazard during the first 90 days and diminished hazard thereafter, you might then have $\beta_1 > 0$ and $\beta_1 + \beta_2 < 0$.

8. Checking the Proportional Hazards Assumption

As pointed out in section 1, the appropriateness of the proportional hazards regression method and the validity of the results depends on the correctness of the proportional hazards assumption given by equation 2. In this section, some graphical and analytic methods of checking on that assumption are discussed. In each case, the check will be for one covariate. Of course, the proportional hazards assumption can be checked separately for each covariate.

Consider first the case of a dichotomous covariate. Let $S_1(t)$ and $S_0(t)$ be the survival functions for the two values of this covariate. As shown in section 4, these functions, under the proportional hazards assumption, are related by $S_1(t) = [S_0(t)]^r$ for some positive number, r. In fact, $r = \exp(\beta)$. Taking natural logarithms of both sides produces

$$\log_e S_1(t) = r \log_e S_0(t) \tag{7}$$

Taking the natural logarithms of the negatives of both sides yields

$$\log_e[-\log_e S_1(t)] = \log_e r + \log_e[-\log_e S_0(t)] \tag{8}$$

According to equation 8, the proportional hazards assumption implies that graphs of $\log_e[-\log_e S_0(t)]$ and $\log_e[-\log_e S_1(t)]$ are parallel. In fact, the constant distance between them should be the coefficient β. You may recall from Chapter 3 that one of the options in PROC LIFETEST is to print graphs of certain functions of the estimated survival function and that $\log_e[-\log_e \hat{S}(t)]$ was one of them. Thus, one way to check on the proportional hazards assumption in this case is to invoke PROC LIFETEST with the dichotomous covariate as a stratification variable and use the option PLOTS = (LLS) or PLOTS = (LOGLOGS). If you have SAS/GRAPH software available, specifying the option GRAPHICS as well will produce a high-resolution graph. Otherwise, you will get cruder line printer plots. You can then inspect the plots visually to see if the curves seem to be separated by a near constant amount. The same approach can be used for a categorical variable with more than two values. The following code shows how this is done for the melanoma data described above and the covariate ULCER.

```
proc lifetest data = melanoma noprint plots = (lls) graphics;
      time dfstime*dfscens(0);
      strata ulcer;
      title 'Figure 4.1';
run;
```

Figure 4.1 shows the graphs of $\log_e[-\log_e \hat{S}_0(t)]$ and $\log_e[-\log_e \hat{S}_1(t)]$ versus $\log_e(t)$ where $\hat{S}_0(t)$ and $\hat{S}_1(t)$ are the Kaplan-Meier estimates of the survival curves for the patients in the melanoma example above with and without ulcers, and t is DFS time. Except for some early (less than $\exp(2) \approx 7$ months) deviation, the graphs are roughly parallel, and the proportional hazards property appears to hold.

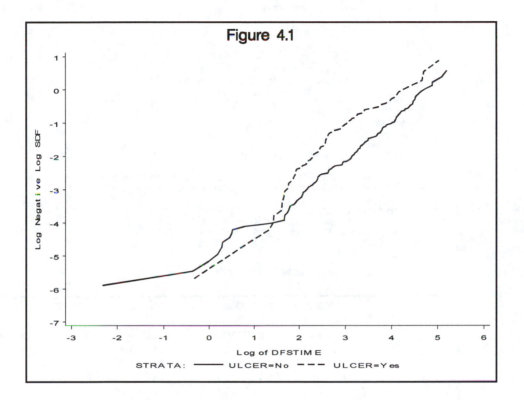

You can also use SAS to calculate $\log_e(-\log_e(S(t)))$ for the two survival functions and to form their differences. The following SAS statements illustrate this approach.

```
/* Get Survival Estimates for Those with Ulcers   */

proc lifetest data = melanoma noprint outs = ulcers   ;
    time dfstime*dfscens(0);
    where ulcer = 1;

/* Get First for Each Month and Calculate log of -log of
 Survival   */

data ulcers;
        set ulcers;
        month = int(dfstime);
proc sort;
        by month dfstime;
data x;
        set ulcers;
        by month;
        if first.month;
        loglogs0= log(-log(survival));
run;
```

```
/* Repeat for Those without Ulcers */

proc lifetest data = melanoma noprint outs = noulcers ;
time dfstime*dfscens(0);
where ulcer = 0;

data noulcers;
      set noulcers;
      month = int(dfstime);
      surv1=survival;
proc sort;
      by month dfstime;
data y;
      set noulcers;
      by month;
      if first.month;
      loglogs1 = log(-log(survival));

/* Merge and Get Differences of log(-log(S)) */

data;
merge x y;
by month;
diff = loglogs1 - loglogs0;

/* Print.  Differences Should be Approximately Constant for
  Proportional Hazards Assumption */

proc print noobs;
var month loglogs1 loglogs0 diff;
where  month in (12 18 24  30 36 42 48);
run;
```

These statements produce the following output:

MONTH	LOGLOGS1	LOGLOGS0	DIFF
12	-2.54483	-1.72520	-0.81962
18	-2.29054	-1.18279	-1.10775
24	-1.96687	-0.87582	-1.09105
30	-1.61257	-0.64472	-0.96785
36	-1.45551	-0.57040	-0.88511
42	-1.32631	-0.47664	-0.84968
48	-1.09288	-0.42166	-0.67122

Note that the differences in the last column are relatively constant.

Another way to use PROC LIFETEST to check on proportional hazards for each group is to specify the lifetable, or actuarial, method of producing survival function estimates, with the same intervals, for each. Then the printed output will include estimates of the hazard at the midpoints of each interval for each group. If proportional hazards hold, their ratio should be relatively constant. Unless the samples are fairly large, the hazard estimates will not be very good, and this method may not work too well.

PROC PHREG itself provides a way to test for certain deviations from proportional hazards. This method is described in the PROC PHREG documentation (SAS Institute, Inc. 1996). Suppose you have a dichotomous (0 or 1) covariate, *group*, for which you want to check the proportional hazards assumption. Define a time dependent covariate by $x(t) = group*t$. The SAS documentation suggests $\log(t)$ instead of t. This avoids numeric problems if the time variable takes on large values — for example, if time is measured in days over several months. Then $x(t)$ is 0 for group 0 and t for group 1. The proportional hazards model based on these two covariates is then

$$h(t,\ group,\ x(t)) = h_0(t)\exp(\beta_1 * group\ +\ \beta_2 * group * t) \tag{7}$$

The risk ratio for group 1 relative to group 2 is $\exp(\beta_1 + \beta_2 t)$. If the estimate of β_2 differs significantly from 0, then that indicates that the risk ratio for group increases (if $\beta_2 > 0$) or decreases (if $\beta_2 < 0$) over time. In either case the risk ratio is not constant.

This test is not a general test of the proportional hazards assumption. It tests the alternative that the hazard ratio changes monotonically over time. If the hazard ratio increases for a while and then decreases, you might not get a statistically significant result for this test.

9. Survival Probabilities

9.1 The BASELINE Statement

As mentioned earlier in this chapter, you are probably more interested in survival probabilities than in hazards. Suppose you use PROC PHREG to establish that higher values of certain covariates and lower values of others are associated with better survival (their beta coefficients are negative and positive respectively). You would next want to know more about the survival probabilities over time for patients with certain specified values of those covariates. PROC PHREG provides such estimated survival probabilities for models in which none of the covariates are time dependent. The technical details underlying the derivation of these estimated survival probabilities are beyond the scope of this book and, for those who are interested, can be found in the PROC PHREG documentation (SAS Institute, Inc. 1996). But it is not necessary to understand those details to obtain the estimates. A typical statement to obtain survival function estimates for specified values of the covariates would look like this:

```
baseline  out=datasetname1  covariates=datasetname2
survival=varname  stderr=varname  lower=varname
    upper = varname;
```

In this statement, *datasetname1* is the name of the SAS data set that will contain the estimates produced. The resultant data set will contain the estimates produced for each value of the time variable in the data set used by PROC PHREG. If it is omitted, SAS uses the DATA*n* convention to assign a name. *Datasetname2* is the name of a SAS data set that you have previously defined. It contains the values of the covariates for which you want survival function estimates. Estimates for the means of the covariates are produced by default. If COVARIATES=*datasetname2* is omitted, only the estimates for the means of the covariates are output to *datasetname1*. The statement above will produce estimates for the survival function, its standard error, and upper and lower bounds for 95% confidence intervals. They will have the variable names specified in the *varname*'s that follow the equal signs. Several other statistics can be calculated in addition to (or instead of) these. Several options can be used after a slash (/). Among them are ALPHA = *value*, which allows you to specify an alpha value other than 0.05 for the (1 – alpha)100% confidence intervals, and NOMEAN, which stops calculation of estimates for the means of the covariates.

9.2 An Example

Consider the melanoma data used previously. Disease-free survival (DFS) is worse for patients with high values of Breslow and Clark and best for patients with low values of those covariates. PROC PHREG will be used with a BASELINE statement to produce survival estimates and their standard errors for three hypothetical patients: one with good anticipated DFS, one with poor anticipated DFS, and an "average" patient. The SAS statements are as follows:

```
data cov_vals;
    input clark breslow;
    cards;
2 .4
4  4
;
PROC PHREG data=melanoma noprint;
    model dfstime*dfscens(0)=breslow clark;
    baseline  covariates=cov_vals  survival=dfs  stderr=se
    lower=lo_bound  upper=up_bound  out=estdfs;
proc print;
run;
```

The results are printed in Output 4.3 below. For each pair of covariate values in the data set COV_VALS, only the first and last twenty lines of the output are reproduced. The lines of output for the mean values of Breslow and Clark are omitted.

Output 4.3

PROC PHREG Survival Function Estimates

OBS	CLARK	BRESLOW	DFSTIME	DFS	SE	LO_BOUND	UP_BOUND
1	2.000	0.400	0.00000	1.00000	.	.	.
2	2.000	0.400	0.00000	0.99915	.0005058	0.99816	1.00000
3	2.000	0.400	0.09868	0.99887	.0005910	0.99771	1.00000
4	2.000	0.400	0.49342	0.99857	.0006717	0.99726	0.99989
5	2.000	0.400	0.62500	0.99828	.0007474	0.99681	0.99974
6	2.000	0.400	0.69079	0.99768	.0008872	0.99595	0.99942
7	2.000	0.400	0.88816	0.99738	.0009536	0.99551	0.99925
8	2.000	0.400	1.21711	0.99707	.0010208	0.99507	0.99908
9	2.000	0.400	1.31579	0.99676	.0010860	0.99464	0.99889
10	2.000	0.400	1.34868	0.99645	.0011499	0.99420	0.99871
11	2.000	0.400	1.64474	0.99613	.0012143	0.99375	0.99851
12	2.000	0.400	1.67763	0.99581	.0012773	0.99331	0.99832
13	2.000	0.400	2.00658	0.99549	.0013404	0.99286	0.99812
14	2.000	0.400	2.17105	0.99516	.0014027	0.99241	0.99791
15	2.000	0.400	2.63158	0.99449	.0015279	0.99150	0.99749

```
16   2.000   0.400   3.68421  0.99415  .0015912   0.99104   0.99728
17   2.000   0.400   3.84868  0.99381  .0016541   0.99057   0.99706
18   2.000   0.400   4.11184  0.99346  .0017174   0.99010   0.99684
19   2.000   0.400   4.67105  0.99311  .0017816   0.98963   0.99661
20   2.000   0.400   4.93421  0.99276  .0018458   0.98914   0.99638


                              .


                              .


                              .
```

```
240  2.000  0.400    90.428  0.70530  0.040076   0.63097   0.78839
241  2.000  0.400    90.559  0.69831  0.040944   0.62250   0.78335
242  2.000  0.400    91.645  0.69123  0.041798   0.61397   0.77820
243  2.000  0.400    93.026  0.68407  0.042658   0.60537   0.77300
244  2.000  0.400    93.355  0.67688  0.043496   0.59678   0.76773
245  2.000  0.400    93.980  0.66883  0.044401   0.58723   0.76177
246  2.000  0.400   102.204  0.65930  0.045656   0.57562   0.75514
247  2.000  0.400   103.618  0.63907  0.048104   0.55141   0.74066
248  2.000  0.400   105.493  0.62839  0.049347   0.53875   0.73295
249  2.000  0.400   109.243  0.61599  0.050787   0.52408   0.72402
250  2.000  0.400   112.829  0.60255  0.052405   0.50812   0.71454
251  2.000  0.400   120.428  0.58675  0.054338   0.48936   0.70353
252  2.000  0.400   129.605  0.56906  0.056534   0.46837   0.69138
253  2.000  0.400   129.638  0.55025  0.058649   0.44651   0.67808
254  2.000  0.400   132.138  0.53009  0.061074   0.42294   0.66439
255  2.000  0.400   151.447  0.50709  0.063899   0.39612   0.64915
256  2.000  0.400   162.138  0.47302  0.068698   0.35584   0.62878
257  2.000  0.400   166.447  0.43531  0.073659   0.31244   0.60649
258  2.000  0.400   178.947  0.37704  0.082897   0.24504   0.58015
259  2.000  0.400   235.559  0.00000  0.000000      .          .
260  4.000  4.000     0.000  1.00000     .          .          .
261  4.000  4.000     0.000  0.99564  0.002517   0.99072   1.00000
262  4.000  4.000     0.099  0.99418  0.002911   0.98849   0.99990
263  4.000  4.000     0.493  0.99269  0.003276   0.98629   0.99913
264  4.000  4.000     0.625  0.99118  0.003609   0.98413   0.99828
265  4.000  4.000     0.691  0.98815  0.004202   0.97995   0.99642
266  4.000  4.000    0.8882  0.98662  0.004475   0.97789   0.99543
267  4.000  4.000    1.2171  0.98505  0.004747   0.97579   0.99439
268  4.000  4.000    1.3158  0.98347  0.005005   0.97371   0.99333
269  4.000  4.000    1.3487  0.98189  0.005254   0.97164   0.99224
270  4.000  4.000    1.6447  0.98027  0.005503   0.96954   0.99112
271  4.000  4.000    1.6776  0.97865  0.005742   0.96746   0.98997
272  4.000  4.000    2.0066  0.97702  0.005977   0.96537   0.98880
273  4.000  4.000    2.1711  0.97537  0.006206   0.96329   0.98761
274  4.000  4.000    2.6316  0.97202  0.006656   0.95907   0.98516
275  4.000  4.000    3.6842  0.97032  0.006880   0.95692   0.98389
```

```
276  4.000  4.000    3.8487 0.96860 0.007098   0.95479   0.98261
277  4.000  4.000    4.1118 0.96687 0.007315   0.95263   0.98131
278  4.000  4.000    4.6711 0.96510 0.007534   0.95045   0.97998
279  4.000  4.000    4.9342 0.96333 0.007748   0.94826   0.97863


                             .

                             .

                             .
```

```
499  4.000  4.000   90.428 0.16626 0.035214   0.10978   0.25181
500  4.000  4.000   90.559 0.15797 0.034754   0.10264   0.24313
501  4.000  4.000   91.645 0.14990 0.034212   0.09584   0.23446
502  4.000  4.000   93.026 0.14210 0.033627   0.08936   0.22596
503  4.000  4.000   93.355 0.13459 0.032970   0.08327   0.21753
504  4.000  4.000   93.980 0.12656 0.032184   0.07689   0.20834
505  4.000  4.000  102.204 0.11757 0.031507   0.06953   0.19879
506  4.000  4.000  103.618 0.10017 0.029670   0.05605   0.17900
507  4.000  4.000  105.493 0.09185 0.028626   0.04987   0.16919
508  4.000  4.000  109.243 0.08291 0.027468   0.04331   0.15872
509  4.000  4.000  112.829 0.07403 0.026279   0.03692   0.14844
510  4.000  4.000  120.428 0.06458 0.024858   0.03037   0.13732
511  4.000  4.000  129.605 0.05518 0.023273   0.02414   0.12612
512  4.000  4.000  129.638 0.04642 0.021404   0.01880   0.11460
513  4.000  4.000  132.138 0.03832 0.019501   0.01414   0.10390
514  4.000  4.000  151.447 0.03051 0.017221   0.01009   0.09224
515  4.000  4.000  162.138 0.02134 0.014175   0.00581   0.07845
516  4.000  4.000  166.447 0.01392 0.011039   0.00294   0.06586
517  4.000  4.000  178.947 0.00665 0.007036   0.00084   0.05287
518  4.000  4.000  235.559 0.00000 0.000000      .         .
```

9.3 Graphs of the Estimated Survival Functions – The Macro PHPLOT

While output such as Output 4.3 provides information about the estimated survival functions for patients with particular covariate values, you would probably like to see this displayed graphically as well. The macro PHPLOT, which is patterned after KMPLOT in Chapter 2, provides graphs of the model-based estimated survival functions. Before using this macro, you should have run PROC PHREG with a BASELINE statement to produce the survival function estimates as described in section 9.2. You must also add a numeric variable taking on the value 1, 2, 3, . . . and so on, to represent the distinct covariate vectors used in the COVARIATES data set. You might also want to provide a label for this variable and a format for its values. This is illustrated in the following example:

```
proc format;
        value c 1 = 'Low' 2 = 'Average' 3 = 'High';
        proc sort data = estdfs;
        by clark breslow;
data estdfs;
        set estdfs;
        by clark breslow time;
        retain c 0;
        if first.breslow then c+1;
        format c c. ;
label c = 'Risk';
```

Now the macro PHPLOT can be invoked. The following template can be used.

```
%phplot(data=         /*Name of dataset to be used.  Default is
                       _LAST_ */
       ,ci=           /*Put confidence intervals on the graphs
                       (yes/no).  Default is no */
       ,yvar=         /*Variable name associatied with keyword
                       survival of baseline statement */
       ,ylabel=       /*Label for vertical axis.  Default is Pct
                       Survival */
       ,byvar=        /*Variable used to distinquish covariate
                       vectors */
       ,xvar=         /*The time variable used in the proc
                       statement. The default is time */
       ,xlabel=       /*The label for the horizontal axis.  The
                       default is Time */
       ,combine=      /*yes to combine curves on one graph, no (the
                       default) to produce seperated graphs for
                       each curve.  If curves are combined on one
                       graph, confidence intervals can not be
                       plotted. */
       ,title=        /*Title to be printed. Default is
                       Proportional Hazards Survival Curve */
       ,lcl=          /*Variable name associated with lower keyword
                       in baseline statement. Default is lcl */
       ,ucl=          /*Variable name associated with upper keyword
                       in baseline statement.  Default is ucl */
)
```

The following example of an invocation of the macro PHPLOT produced Figure 4.2:

```
%phplot(
       yvar=dfs             /*Variable name associated with
                             keyword survival of baseline
                             statement */
       ,ylabel=Pct DFS      /*Label for vertical axis.  Default is
                             Pct Survival */
       ,byvar=c             /*Variable used to distinquish covariate
                             vectors */
       ,xvar=dfstime        /*The time variable used in the proc
                             statement. The default is time */
       ,xlabel=Months       /*The label for the horizontal axis.
                             The default is Time */
       ,combine= yes        /*yes to combine curves on one graph, no
                             (the default) to produce seperate
                             graphs for each curve.  If curves are
                             combined on one graph, confidence
                             intervals can not be plotted. */
       ,title = Figure 4.2  /*Title to be printed. Default is
                             Proportional Hazards Survival Curve */
       ,lcl = lo_bound      /*Variable name associated with lower
                             keyword in baseline statement.
                             Default is lcl */
       ,ucl = up_bound      /*Variable name associated with upper
                             keyword in baseline statement.
                             Default is ucl */
)
```

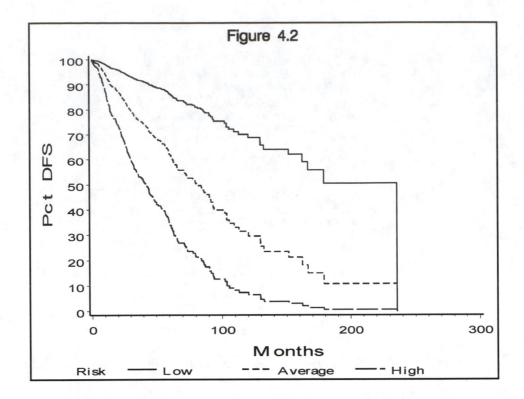

Figure 4.2

10. Power and Sample Size

10.1 The Nature of the Problem

Turning to the issues of power and sample size, there are two related questions that can be asked:

1. How large a sample do you need to ensure a specified power for a test of a null hypothesis that one of the beta coefficients is 0?

2. Given a sample of a given size, what is the power for the test of a null hypothesis that one of the beta coefficients is 0?

The first type of question should be answered when you are planning a study. The second is relevant when you are given an existing set of data to analyze. In particular, if you find that a beta coefficient estimate is not signicantly different from 0, you might want to know if there was much probability of getting a significant result, even for meaningful values of the beta coefficient, with the available sample. The macro PHPOW, described in section 10.3, addresses both types of questions.

In thinking about the nature of the proportional hazards model, it is clear that a general approach to these problems is not practical. There are just too many sources of complexity. In order to say anything about power or sample size for the general model, you would need to specify the beta coefficients of all of the covariates. In addition, the joint distribution of the covariates in the population from which the sample is drawn would have to be specified. Finally, the underlying hazard function, $h_0(t)$ would affect the calculations as well.

10.2 The Lui Method

The method implemented by PHPOW is based on an article by Lui (1992) which deals with a highly restricted, yet useful, proportional hazards model. Consider a proportional hazards model with two dichotomous covariates, x_1, and x_2. Assume that each takes on the values 0 and 1. Suppose that x_1 is the covariate of interest and x_2 is a confounder. For example, x_1 might be the treatment group to which the patient was assigned, and x_2 might be a factor thought to impact on survival, perhaps the existence or non-existence of a particular form of comorbidity. Let β_1 and β_2 be the associated beta coefficients. The joint distribution can be expressed by the numbers p_{ij} for i and j each being 0 or 1. Each p_{ij} is the probability that x_1 is i and x_2 is j. Since these numbers must sum to 1.0, any three of them determine the fourth. If patients are randomized with equal allocation to groups (determined by the covariate of interest) 0 or 1, then $p_{00} + p_{01} = p_{10} + p_{11} = 0.5$, $p_{00} = p_{10}$, and $p_{01} = p_{11}$. The following method allows for non-random assignment as well. Furthermore, suppose that the underlying hazard function is the constant λ. Thus, the survival function is exponential with possibly different hazards for different values of x_1 and x_2. Specifically,

$$S(t, x_1, x_2) = \exp[-\lambda(e^{\beta_1 x_1 + \beta_2 x_2})t] \qquad (9)$$

Let t be the accrual time and τ be the post-accrual follow-up period. You intend to test the null hypothesis that $\beta_1 = 0$ against the two-sided alternative that $\beta_1 \neq 0$ at significance level α.

10.3 The PHPOW Macro

The formula given by Lui requires the user to provide values for p_{00}, p_{01}, p_{10}, $t, \tau, \beta_1, \beta_2$, λ, and α. Since it is more natural to think in terms of survival probabilities than hazards, the macro PHPOW allows you to provide survival probabilities at some convenient times for three groups of patients: S_{00} for those with $x_1 = x_2 = 0$; S_{01} for those with $x_1 = 0$ and $x_2 = 1$; and S_{10} for those with $x_1 = 1$ and $x_2 = 0$ instead. PHPOW uses these values to calculate values for $\beta_1, \beta_2, \lambda$. In keeping with the two types of questions above, you can provide a value for the desired power or sample size. The macro, which is given at the end of this chapter, calculates the value that you do not provide. The following template can be used to invoke the macro.

```
%macro phpow(
            p00=              /* Proportion with x1=0, x2=0 */
           ,p01=              /* Proportion with x1=0, x2=1 */
           ,p10=              /* Proportion with x1=1, x2=0 */
           ,s00=              /* A survival probability for
                                 x1=x2=0 */
           ,t00=              /* The time associated with s00 */
           ,s01=              /* A survival probability for x1=0,
                                 x2=1 */
           ,t01=              /* The time associated with s01 */
           ,s10=              /* A survival probability for x1=1,
                                 x2=0 */
           ,t10=              /* The time associated with s10 */
           ,t=                /* Accrual time */
           ,tau=              /* Post accrual follow-up */
           ,alpha=            /* Significance level of test.
                                 Default is 0.05 */
           ,power=            /* Power of test. (optional)
           ,n=                /* Sample Size.  (optional) Note:
                                 power or n, but not both, must be
                                 given */
)
```

10.4 An Example

Suppose you are planning a study to compare an experimental treatment ($x_1 = 1$) to standard treatment ($x_1 = 0$). It is known that 70% of those in the study population are men ($x_2 = 0$) and that they tend to do worse than women ($x_2 = 1$). Data based on the standard treatment indicate three-year survival of 50% among men and 70% among women. Thus $S_{00} = 0.5$ and $S_{01} = 0.7$. Since the treatment is to be assigned randomly with equal allocation to each, we have $p_{00} = p_{10} = 0.35$ and $p_{01} = 0.15$. You plan to accrue for five years and to follow patients for three years after accrual ends. You would like to have 80% power for a test of $\beta_1 = 0$ if the experimental treatment improves three-year survival among men to 65%. That means that $S_{10} = .65$. Of course, we have $t_{00} = t_{01} = t_{10} = 3$. The macro PHPOW is invoked by this statement

```
%phpow(
            p00=0.35          /* Proportion with x1=0, x2=0 */
           ,p01=0.15          /* Proportion with x1=0, x2=1   */
           ,p10=0.35          /* Proportion with x1=1, x2=0 */
           ,s00=0.5           /* A survival probability for
                                 x1=x2=0 */
           ,t00=3             /* The time associated with s00 */
           ,s01=0.7           /* A survival probability for x1=0,
                                 x2=1 */
           ,t01=3             /* The time associated with s01 */
           ,s10=0.65          /* A survival probability for x1=1,
                                 x2=0 */
           ,t10=3             /* The time associated with s10 */
           ,t=5               /* Accrual time */
           ,tau=3             /* Post accrual follow-up */
           ,power=0.8         /* Power of test. (optional) */
           ,n=                /* Sample Size.  (optional) Note:  power
                                 or n but not both, must be given */
)
```

Here are results, showing that 230 patients will be needed:

Results of PHPOW								
OBS P00 P01 P10 P11					B1	B2	ALPHA	POWER N
1 0.35 0.15 0.35 0.15					-0.47564	-0.66442	0.05	0.8 230

Note that the beta coefficients calculated from the given survival probabilities are also given. Thus, those probabilities are seen to imply hazard ratios of $\exp(-0.47564) = 0.62$ for the experimental treatment relative to the standard (under the alternative hypothesis) and $\exp(-0.66442) = 0.51$ for females relative to males.

11. Additional Details

11.1 An Introduction to Likelihood-Based Estimation and Inference

The general situation is that a survival, hazard, or density function of a certain type is assumed for a population. You saw in Chapter 1 that, given any one of these, you can, at least theoretically, obtain the others. Suppose that function has one or more parameters whose values are not known. The problem is to estimate them from a sample taken at random from the population. There are often many ways that this can be done, but with all estimation methods, you should keep in mind these three considerations:

1.   There should be some logical basis for the method of estimation. That is, the estimate should be a number that uniquely fits some reasonable criterion.

2.   The criterion of item 1 should lead to a method of calculation that we can do. Of course, that method might be practical only with a computer. But that is fine.

3.   Since the estimate is the result of calculations on a random sample, it is itself a random variable. It would be nice to know something about the distribution of that random variable in order to perform statistical inferences and produce confidence intervals. In many cases it can be shown that an estimate is approximately, for large samples, normally distributed with mean equal to the parameter being estimated and a variance that can be estimated from the data. This makes it possible to create a confidence interval for the parameter and to perform tests of hypotheses. This topic will be explored in detail later in this section.

Start with a very simple example. Assume that a population has exponential survival. From Chapter 1, that means that the density function of survival time is of the form $f(t, \lambda) = \lambda \exp(-\lambda t)$ for some positive number, λ, that you would like to estimate and for $0 \le t < \infty$. The parameter, λ, is included on the left side to remind us that the density depends on λ. Generally, you would want a larger sample, but suppose you want to estimate λ based on a sample of one patient who died at time $t = 3$ years. What is a reasonable way to estimate the parameter based on this data?

Consider a small time interval of width Δt containing $t = 3$. As seen in Chapter 1, the probability that a patient's death will be in that interval is approximately $f(3, \lambda)\Delta t$. Since the patient did die in that interval of time, a reasonable approach would be to estimate λ by a number that makes that probability as large as possible. That is, estimate λ by a value that maximizes the probability of the occurrence of an event that we know did occur. But $f(3, \lambda)\Delta t$ is maximized by maximizing $f(3, \lambda)$, which is $\lambda \exp(-3\lambda)$; so we should, by this criterion, choose the value of λ that maximizes the value of the density with t fixed at its observed value.

The problem now is to maximize $\lambda\exp(-3\lambda)$. How do you do that? First of all, note that the value of the parameter that maximizes a function is the same value that maximizes its natural logarithm. Often, in problems like this, the natural logarithm is easier to deal with. So concentrate on maximizing $\log_e(\lambda) - 3\lambda$ instead. Of course, you could get a good idea of the value of λ that maximizes $\log_e(\lambda) - 3\lambda$ by calculating its value for a large number of values of λ. However, elementary calculus provides a better approach. Often, although not always, a function is maximized by the value at which its derivative is 0. This leads to solving the equation $1/\lambda - 3 = 0$. The solution is $\frac{1}{3}$. The function $f(3, \lambda)$ is called a *likelihood*, its natural logarithm is called a *loglikelihood*, and $\frac{1}{3}$ is called the *maximum likelihood estimator* (MLE) of λ. It is common to denote the MLE of a parameter by the symbol for the parameter with a "hat." Thus you can write $\hat{\lambda} = \frac{1}{3}$.

Extending this concept to random samples of size greater than 1 is not difficult. Again consider, as an example, the exponential model above. This time though, you have a sample with survival times $t_1, t_2, \ldots, t_n$. Since the probability that n independent events all happen is the product of the probabilities of each of the individual events, the function to be maximized is now

$$\prod_{i=1}^{n} \lambda\exp(-\lambda t_i) = \lambda^n\exp\left(-\lambda\sum_{i=1}^{n} t_i\right) \tag{10}$$

Taking the natural logarithm, you need to maximize

$$n\log_e(\lambda) - \lambda\sum_{i=1}^{n} t_i \tag{11}$$

Equating the derivative with respect to λ to zero yields the equation

$$\frac{n}{\lambda} - \sum_{i=1}^{n} t_i = 0 \tag{12}$$

The solution, $n/\sum_{i=1}^{n} t_i$, is the MLE, $\hat{\lambda}$. You should realize that in many situations the equation to be solved is more complex than equation 12. Often, such situations require numeric approximation methods that would be very tedious without a computer.

You are probably surprised that this discussion completely ignores censored data. That omission is easily rectified. If a survival time, t_i, is censored, then its probability is simply $S(t_i, \lambda)$. Thus, that factor is used instead of $f(t_i, \lambda)$ in forming the likelihood. For the exponential model, if the data consist of n pairs of the form (t_i, d_i) for $i = 1, \ldots, n$, where $d_i = 0$ for a censored observation and 1 for a complete observation, the likelihood becomes

$$\prod_{i=1}^{n} \lambda^{d_i} \exp(-\lambda t_i) = \lambda^{\sum_{i=1}^{n} d_i} \exp(-\lambda \sum_{i=1}^{n} t_i) \tag{13}$$

The natural logarithm of equation 13 is $D\log_e(\lambda) - \lambda \sum_{i=1}^{n} t_i$ where D is the number of uncensored times. Setting the derivative with respect to λ,

$\dfrac{D}{\lambda} - \sum_{i=1}^{n} t_i$, equal to 0 and solving for λ, then the following solution

is the MLE of λ, $\hat{\lambda}$: $\dfrac{D}{\sum_{i=1}^{n} t_i}$

To generalize the above discussion to arbitrary survival distributions with one parameter, θ, let $S(t, \theta)$ and $f(t, \theta)$ be the survival and density functions, respectively. Suppose θ is to be estimated from the data (t_i, d_i) for $i = 1, \ldots, n$ as described above. Let

$$L(\theta) = \prod_{d_i=0} S(t_i, \theta) \prod_{d_i=1} f(t_i, \theta) \tag{14}$$

and

$$\log_e L(\theta) = \sum_{d_i=0} \log_e[S(t_i, \theta)] + \sum_{d_i=1} \log_e[f(t_i, \theta)] \tag{15}$$

Then the maximum likelihood estimator of θ is the value that maximizes the likelihood, $L(\theta)$, or equivalently, the loglikelihood, $\log_e L(\theta)$. Often, this value is found as the solution of $d\log_e L(\theta)/d\theta = 0$.

It is not hard to extend these ideas to more than one parameter. Suppose there are K parameters, $\theta_1, \theta_2, \ldots, \theta_K$. Let θ be the column vector, $(\theta_1, \theta_2, \ldots, \theta_K)'$. The density function and survival function can be written as $f(t, \theta)$ and $S(t, \theta)$ respectively. The loglikelihood becomes

$$\log_e L(\theta) = \sum_{d_i=0} \log_e[S(t_i, \theta)] + \sum_{d_i=1} \log_e[f(t_i, \theta)] \tag{16}$$

The MLE of θ, which will be denoted $\hat{\theta}$, is the vector of values for $\theta_1, \theta_2, \ldots, \theta_K$ that maximizes equation 16. These values can often be found as the simultaneous solution of the system of equations formed by equating the partial derivatives of $\log_e L(\theta)$ to 0. This is generally a problem for a computer and a specialized program. As you will see in Chapter 5, SAS has facilities that can make the maximization of a loglikelihood fairly easy.

Turning to issues of inferences about the parameters, there are two properties that are very useful in this regard. The first concerns the distribution of the vector $\hat{\theta} = (\hat{\theta}_1, \hat{\theta}_2, \ldots, \hat{\theta}_K)$. Under fairly mild conditions, as the sample size increases, that vector has approximately a multivariate normal distribution with mean vector equal to $(\theta_1, \theta_2, \ldots, \theta_K)$. The covariance matrix of $\hat{\theta} = (\hat{\theta}_1, \hat{\theta}_2, \ldots, \hat{\theta}_K)$ can be approximated by considering the matrix in which the row i column j element is the second partial derivative, $\partial^2 \ln L(\theta)/\partial\theta_i\partial\theta_j$. This matrix, denoted $\mathbf{I}$, is often called Fisher's Information Matrix. Letting $\mathbf{V} = -\mathbf{I}^{-1}$, $\mathbf{V}$ is the approximate covariance matrix of $(\hat{\theta}_1, \hat{\theta}_2, \ldots, \hat{\theta}_K)$. The j'th diagonal entry, v_{jj}, is the approximate variance of the estimate $\hat{\theta}_j$. Thus, for any parameter, θ_j, $\hat{\theta}_j \pm z_{\alpha/2} v_{jj}^{1/2}$ is an approximate $(1-\alpha)100\%$ confidence interval for θ_j. In PROC PHREG, where the risk ratios are the $\exp(\theta_j)$, $(1-\alpha)100\%$ confidence intervals for these risk ratios can be written as $\exp(\hat{\theta}_j \pm z_{\alpha/2} v_{jj}^{1/2})$. It also follows that, under the null hypothesis of $\theta_j = 0$, $\hat{\theta}_j^2/v_{jj}$ has a χ^2 distribution with one degree of freedom. This statistic is what is called the Wald Chi-Square in the PROC PHREG output. Another important consequence of the normality of the estimated vector of parameters is that $\hat{\theta}'\mathbf{V}^{-1}\hat{\theta}$ has, under the null hypothesis that all of the parameters are 0, a χ^2 distribution with $K-1$ degrees of freedom. This is seen as the Wald criterion, one of the three tests of the global null hypothesis in the PROC PHREG output. It is also called the Residual Chi-square in each model selection step.

For another approach to hypothesis testing involving maximum likelihood, consider a null hypothesis that assigns specific values to certain parameters, say m of them, where $0 < m \leq K$. As above, let $\hat{\theta}$ be the MLE of the vector of parameters, θ. Let $\hat{\theta}_0$ be the MLE of θ restricted by the null hypothesis. That is, the m parameters of the null hypothesis have their specified values, and the other $K-m$ parameters have the values that maximize the likelihood subject to that restriction. Now consider the ratio $L(\hat{\theta})/L(\hat{\theta}_0)$. The numerator must be greater than or equal to the denominator because it maximizes the likelihood over a larger set of values. If the fraction is near 1, that indicates that the sample observed was almost as "likely" with the restriction of the null hypothesis as it is without that restriction. This would argue for the reasonableness of the null hypothesis.

On the other hand, if the ratio is large, you would feel that the null hypothesis is not too reasonable and be more inclined to reject it. Likelihood ratio tests are a class of statistical tests that reject the null hypothesis for sufficiently large values of the ratio $L(\hat{\theta})/L(\hat{\theta}_0)$. Many familiar statistical tests, although they may not be presented this way, are actually likelihood ratio tests. Among them are the familiar (pooled and paired) t-tests and one-way ANOVA. The trick, of course, is to determine the distribution of the likelihood ratio under the null hypothesis. Then, for a desired significance level, α, you can choose a critical value c such that the probability, under the null hypothesis, that $L(\hat{\theta})/L(\hat{\theta}_0) > c$ is α. It follows that we would reject the null hypothesis if $L(\hat{\theta})/L(\hat{\theta}_0) > c$.

In many cases, however, determination of the distribution of $L(\hat{\theta})/L(\hat{\theta}_0)$ under the null hypothesis is not feasible. In such cases, an approximation that holds as the size of the sample increases is useful. That approximation is that $2\log_e[L(\hat{\theta})/L(\hat{\theta}_0)]$ has a distribution that, under the null hypothesis, is approximately χ^2 with m degrees of freedom. Thus, the null hypothesis is rejected if $2\log_e[L(\hat{\theta})/L(\hat{\theta}_0)]$ exceeds a critical value chosen from the distribution of the χ^2 distribution with m degrees of freedom. A special case of interest is when $m = K$; that is, the null hypothesis specifies values for all of the parameters. Then the denominator, $L(\hat{\theta}_0)$, of the likelihood ratio is just $L(\theta_0)$, the value of the likelihood with all of the parameters given their specified values. This is the statistic used as one of the tests of the global null hypothesis as the "$-2 \log L$" criterion.

Another statistic used with likelihood-based inference is called the *score statistic*. Use the notation, $\mathbf{0}$, to represent a vector in which each component is 0. Let $\partial\log_e L(\mathbf{0})/\partial\theta$ be the column vector in which the j'th component is the partial derivative of $\log_e L(\theta)$ with respect to θ_j evaluated with each $\theta_j = 0$. Let $\partial^2\log_e L(\mathbf{0})/\partial\theta^2$ be the matrix in which the row i, column j component is the second partial derivative $\partial^2\log_e L(\theta)/\partial\theta_i\partial\theta_j$ evaluated with each $\theta_j = 0$. Then the score statistic for the null hypothesis that all of the parameters are 0 is defined by

$$[\partial\mathbf{log_e L(0)}/\partial\theta]'[-\partial^2\mathbf{log_e L(0)}/\partial\theta^2]^{-1}[\partial\mathbf{log_e L(0)}/\partial\theta] \qquad (17)$$

That statistic has, under the null hypothesis, an approximate χ^2 distribution with K degrees of freedom. The score statistic is used as one of the three tests of the global null hypothesis.

11.2 Partial Likelihood and the Proportional Hazards Model

If you were to attempt to use the likelihood methods described above for the proportional hazards model of this chapter, you would run into an immediate problem. In addition to the beta parameters, that model has an underlying hazard function that would need to be estimated as well. The contribution of the classic paper by Cox (1972) is to condition the likelihood on the ordering of the complete and censored observations. This results in what is called a partial likelihood, in which the underlying hazard is not a factor.

Let the data be represented by the triples $(t_i, d_i, \mathbf{x}_i)$ for $i = 1, 2, \ldots, n$ where t_i is the observation time, $d_i = 0$ (censored) or 1 (uncensored), and $\mathbf{x}_i$ is a column vector of covariate values for the i'th patient. For now, assume no tied times so that all of the t_i are distinct. To simplify the notation below, let the times be ordered so that $t_1 < t_2 < \ldots < t_n$. Now consider a particular time t_i for which $d_i = 1$ so that a death occurred at time t_i. By the definition equation 2 of the proportional hazards model, the probability of that death within an interval of width Δt containing t_i is approximately

$$h_0(t_i)\exp(\beta'\mathbf{x}_i)\Delta t_i \qquad (18)$$

But all of the patients who were observed for time t_i or more, that is with time t_j where $j \geq i$, had similar probabilities of dying in that interval (with $\mathbf{x}_i$ replaced by $\mathbf{x}_j$ and t_i replaced by t_j). Thus the probability that one of them died in that interval is approximately

$$\sum_{j \geq i} h_0(t_i)\exp(\beta'\mathbf{x}_j)\Delta t_i \tag{19}$$

To form an estimate of the conditional probability of the death of the patient whose observation time was t_i given that there was a death among those observed for at least that long, divide the probability given by equation 18 by the probability given by equation 19. Then taking the product of all such quotients over all deaths yields

$$\prod_{d_i=1} \frac{\exp(\beta'\mathbf{x}_i)}{\sum\limits_{j \geq i} \exp(\beta'\mathbf{x}_j)} \tag{20}$$

Now, what if ties are allowed? Then d_i can represent the number of deaths at time t_i. The numerator is then derived from the product of the probabilities of each of the d_i deaths. But this can be obtained by simply adding the exponents. In other words, $\mathbf{x}_i$ can be replaced by $\mathbf{s}_i$, the sum of the covariate vectors for the patients who died at time t_i. For the denominator, the probability of d_i deaths at time t_i is approximately the denominator in equation 20 raised to the d_i power.

The final result is what is known as the partial likelihood, given by

$$\prod_{d_i \geq 1} \frac{\exp(\beta's_i)}{[\sum\limits_{j \geq i} \exp(\beta'\mathbf{x}_j)]^{d_i}} \tag{21}$$

PROC PHREG uses the Newton-Raphson iterative procedure to find the vector β that maximizes equation 21. While that expression is not a true likelihood, it has been shown that the resultant estimate has the properties described above.

For a stratified analysis, the products of the form in equation 21 are created separately for each level of the stratification variable. This allows for different underlying hazard functions for different strata. The likelihood to be maximized is the product of the partial likelihoods over the strata.

11.3 The PHPLOT Macro

```
%macro phplot(data =       , ci=no, yvar=survival,
              ylabel=Pct Survival, byvar= none,
              xvar=time,xlabel=Time,combine=no,
              title='Proportional Hazards Survival Curve',
              lcl=lcl, ucl = ucl );

/* Symbol statements for up to 4 curves on one graph */

%if &combine=yes %then %do;
        %let ci=no;
symbol1 l=1  v=none  i=stepjl w=5;
symbol2 l=3 v=none i=stepjl w=5;
symbol3 l=5 v=none i=stepjl w=5;
symbol4 l=33 v=none i=stepjl w=5;
%end;

/* Symbol Statements for separate graphs */

%if &combine=no %then %do;
symbol1 l=1  v= none i=stepjl w=5;
symbol2 l=3 v=none i=stepjl w=5;
symbol3 l=3 v=none i=stepjl w=5;
%end;

%if &byvar=none %then goptions cby=white;;
data;
        set &data;
        survival=&yvar*100;
        lcl=100*&lcl;
        ucl=100*&ucl;
        y=survival;
        curve=1;
        output;
        y=ucl;
        curve=2;
        %if &ci=yes %then output;;
        y=lcl;
        curve=3;
        %if &ci=yes %then output;;
proc sort;
        by &byvar curve &xvar;
run;
proc format;
value curve 1='PH curve'
              2='UCL'
              3='LCL';
axis1 width=5 minor=none label=(h=2 f=swiss a=90 j=center
   "&ylabel")value=(h=1.5 f=swiss) order=(0 to 100 by 10);
axis2 width=5 label=(h=2 f=swiss  "&xlabel") value=(h=1.5
     f=swiss);
%if &combine=no %then legend1 label=(f=swiss h=1.5  'Curve')
                                value=(f=swiss h=1.5 j=1
                                'PH Curve' "UCL" "LCL");;
legend2 label=(f=swiss h=1.5) value=(f=swiss h=1.5 j=1);

/* PROC GPLOT for separate graphs */
%if &combine=no %then %do;
proc gplot;
        plot y*&xvar= curve /
        legend=legend1
        vaxis=axis1 haxis=axis2
        %if &ci=no %then nolegend;;
        ;
        by &byvar;
        format curve curve.;
        %end;
```

```
/* PROC GPLOT for combined graphs */

%if &combine=yes %then %do;
        proc gplot;
        plot y*&xvar=&byvar/ legend=legend2
        vaxis=axis1 haxis=axis2;
        %end;
title &title;
run;
%mend phplot;
```

11.4 The PHPOW Macro

```
/*  This is a macro for calculating the sample size needed for a
    proportional hazards regression with two dichotomous
    covariates, x1 and x2.  x1 is the covariate of interest and
    x2 is the confounder.  The macro is based on Lui(1992),
    Controlled Clinical Trials, 13:446-458 */

%macro phpow(p00=  , p01= , p10=  ,s00= ,t00= ,s01=, t01=,
             s10= ,t10=, t= , tau=  , alpha= .05  ,power= , n= );
data;
/* Convert from macro variables to numeric */

        alpha = symget('alpha') + 0;
        power = symget('power') + 0;
        n=symget('n');
        p00 = symget('p00') + 0;
        p01 = symget('p01') + 0;
        p10 = symget('p10') + 0;
        t = symget('t') + 0;
        tau = symget('tau') + 0;
        s00 = symget('s00') + 0;
        s01 = symget('s01') + 0;
        t00 = symget('t00') + 0;
        t01 = symget('t01') + 0;
        s10 = symget('s10') + 0;
        t10 = symget('t10') + 0;
/* Calculate other values that are needed */

        zalpha = -probit(alpha/2);
        zbeta = probit(power);
        p11 = 1 - p00 - p01 - p10;
        lambda = -log(s00)/t00;
        b1 = log(-log(s10)/(lambda*t10));
        b2 = log(-log(s01)/(lambda*t01));
        t0=t + tau;
        p0plus = p00 + p01;
        p1plus = 1 - p0plus;
        pplus0 = p10 + p00;
        pplus1 = 1 - pplus0;
        phi = (p11*p00 - p10*p01)/sqrt(p1plus*p0plus*pplus1*pplus0);

/*  Using formula 3, page 448 and formula 5, 449 */

/*  Alternative b1 */

        a1=(1+(exp(-lambda*t0)-exp(-lambda*tau))/(lambda*t))*p00
           +(1+(exp(-lambda*t0*exp(b1))-
           exp(-lambda*tau*exp(b1)))/lambda*t*exp(b1)))*p10+
           (1+(exp(-lambda*t0*exp(b2))-exp(-lambda*tau*exp(b2))))/
           (lambda*t*exp(b2)))*p01+(1+(exp(-lambda*t0*exp(b1+
           b2))-exp(-lambda*tau*exp(b1+b2))))/
           (lambda*t*exp(b1+b2)))*p11;

/* Null hypothesis b1 = 0 */

        a0=(1+(exp(-lambda*t0)-exp(-lambda*tau))/(lambda*t))*p00
           +(1+(exp(-lambda*t0)-exp(-lambda*tau))/(lambda*t))*p10
           +(1+(exp(-lambda*t0*exp(b2))-exp(-lambda*tau*exp(b2))))/
           (lambda*t*exp(b2)))*p01+(1+(exp(-lambda*t0*exp(b2))-
           exp(-lambda*tau*exp(b2)))/lambda*t*exp(b2)))*p11;
```

```
/*   Under alternative b1 */

        q00=(1 + (exp(-lambda*t0)-exp(-lambda*tau))
            /(lambda*t))/a1*p00;
        q10=(1 + (exp(-lambda*t0*exp(b1))-
            exp(-lambda*tau*exp(b1)))/(lambda*t*exp(b1)))/a1*p10;
        q01=(1+(exp(-lambda*t0*exp(b2))-exp(-lambda*tau*exp(b2)))/
            (lambda*t*exp(b2)))/a1*p01;
        q11=(1+(exp(-lambda*t0*exp(b1+b2))-exp(-lambda*tau*
            exp(b1+b2)))/(lambda*t*exp(b1+b2)))/a1*p11;
        q0plus=q00+q01;
        q1plus=q10+q11;
        qplus0=q10+q00;
        qplus1=q01+q11;
        phistar=(q11*q00-q10*q01)/sqrt(q1plus*q0plus*qplus1*qplus0);
        v1=(a1*q1plus*(1-q1plus)*(1-phistar**2))**(-1);

/*   Under null hypothesis, b1 = 0   */

q00=(1+(exp(-lambda*t0)-exp(-lambda*tau))/(lambda*t))/a0*p00;

q10=(1+(exp(-lambda*t0)-exp(-lambda*tau))/(lambda*t))/a0*p10;
    q01=(1+(exp(-lambda*t0*exp(b2))-exp(-lambda*tau*exp(b2)))/
        (lambda*t*exp(b2)))/a0*p01;
        q11=(1+(exp(-lambda*t0*exp(b2))-exp(-lambda*tau*exp(b2)))/
            (lambda*t*exp(b2)))/a0*p11;
        q0plus=q00+q01;
        q1plus=q10+q11;
        qplus0=q10+q00;
        qplus1=q01+q11;
        phistar=(q11*q00-q10*q01)/sqrt(q1plus*q0plus*qplus1*qplus0);
        v0=(a0*q1plus*(1-q1plus)*(1-phistar**2))**(-1);
        if n=. then n=int((zalpha*sqrt(v0)+
                    zbeta*sqrt(v1))**2/b1**2)+1;
if power= . then power=probnorm((sqrt(n*b1**2)-
                    zalpha*sqrt(v0))/sqrt(v1));
proc print;
        var p00 p01 p10 p11 b1 b2 alpha power n;
run;
%mend;
```

Chapter 5 Parametric Methods

1. Introduction

In this chapter, a process that was begun in Chapter 2 is brought to a logical conclusion.
In that chapter and in Chapter 3, you were introduced to methods of survival analysis that
made no assumptions about the underlying survival distribution(s). Such methods are
said to be nonparametric. In Chapter 4, certain assumptions about the nature of the
hazard function were made for the proportional hazards regression method. Since the
underlying hazard is left unspecified, this method is called semi-parametric. In this
chapter, the next step is taken. It is assumed that the survival function is of a certain
form, such as exponential, Weibull, etc., with one or more parameters whose values are
unknown. The idea, of course, is to estimate those values from a set of survival data.
These estimates, then, complete the specification of the survival function.

Two approaches to this problem are presented. The first is to use the LIFEREG
procedure. This procedure is based on a model known as the *accelerated failure time
model*. It allows for the specification of a vector of covariates and provides information

about the effect of these covariates on survival times. In this sense it resembles the PHREG procedure, which was discussed in Chapter 4. You will see, however, that the effect of a covariate in this model is quite different from that of the proportional hazards model. Because of the model used, this method requires the assumption of one of five types of survival functions. The second approach is to use a macro, PARAMEST, which is described later in this chapter. This macro allows you to specify any survival function with any number of parameters. Estimates of the values of the parameters are produced. Explanatory covariates are permitted in this macro as well. Using the macro PARAMEST is a bit more difficult than using PROC LIFEREG. It is necessary to specify both the survival distribution and the hazard function as functions of the parameters and time. In addition, the use of this macro requires more computer time. However, it does permit greater flexibility in the specification of the underlying distribution and the effects of the covariates.

Both of these parametric approches have an important feature not found in the methods presented previously. They both allow for right-censored, left-censored, or interval-censored data. A survival time is left censored if what is known about it is that it is no more than a value, t. A survival time is interval censored if what is known about it is that it is at least some value, say t_1, and less than some greater value, t_2. Interval censoring is fairly common. If patients are followed periodically for recurrence of disease, one might be disease free when checked at time t_1 but have the disease when checked at a later time t_2. If you don't know when the disease recurred, but only that it was between t_1 and t_2, then the recurrence time is interval censored by the interval (t_1, t_2). When using methods that do not allow for interval censoring, analysts generally define the event time to be the time at which the event was first observed. Thus, an investigator checking for the event annually will, all other factors being equal, tend to report longer times than an investigator checking for the event every six months. The ability to deal with interval censoring is an important feature of the methods of this chapter. Left censoring is less common. In the above situation, patients found to have recurred at the time of their first follow-up visit would be left censored. Of course, left censoring can be thought of as interval censoring with the left endpoint of the censoring interval being 0. In order for PROC LIFEREG or the macro PARAMEST to deal with these forms of censoring, the data set must convey the necessary information. This is accomplished by having two time variables in the data set, say t_1 and t_2. The roles of t_1 and t_2 are described as follows:

If . . .	Then ...
t_2 is a missing value	t_1 is considered a right-censored time
t_1 is a missing value	t_2 is considered a left-censored time
neither t_1 nor t_2 is a missing value and $t_1 < t_2$	time is considered censored in the interval (t_1, t_2)
$t_1 = t_2$ and not a missing value	time is complete with the common value

Consider, for example, the following data:

PATID	t1	t2
1	.	7.8
2	2.3	5.9
3	4.6	.
4	7.3	7.3

Patient #1 had the event occur sometime prior to time 7.8. Patient #2 had the event occur between times 2.3 and 5.9. Patient #3 was event-free at time 4.6. Patient #4 had the event occur at time 7.3. The fact that the form of the survival function is specified allows for the accommodation of these forms of censoring.

2. The Accelerated Failure Time Model

You are probably already familiar with the linear regression model presented in most elementary statistics texts. The basic assumption is that a dependent variable, y, is related to a set of independent variables, $x_1, x_2, \ldots, x_k$ by a relationship of the form $y = \beta_0 + \beta_1 x_1 + \ldots + \beta_k x_k + \sigma \varepsilon$ where $\beta_0, \beta_1, \ldots, \beta_k$ are unknown regression coefficients, ε is a random variable having a standard normal distribution, and σ is a positive number. You might wonder whether this approach would work with y replaced by survival time. That could be done. But since survival time cannot be negative, it is more common to use the natural logarithm of the survival time as the dependent variable. Also, in addition to the standard normal distribution, the random variable ε can be assumed to have other distributions as well. Of course, the distribution chosen for ε determines the distribution of survival time. In the following discussion, T will represent the random survival time, and Y its natural logarithm. Assume that, for each patient, k covariates, $x_1, x_2, \ldots, x_k$ are observed. Let ε be a random variable. Then, the accelerated failure time model implies that for some set of coefficients $\beta_0, \beta_1, \ldots, \beta_k$ and positive number, σ, we have

$$Y = \beta_0 + \beta_1 x_1 \ldots \beta_k x_k + \sigma \varepsilon$$

or equivalently

$$T = \exp(\beta_0 + \beta_1 x_1 + \ldots \beta_k x_k + \sigma \varepsilon) \tag{1}$$

The parameters β_0 and σ are called the intercept and scale parameters. The parameters $\beta_1, \ldots, \beta_k$ describe the way that survival time is affected by the values of the covariates. A value of 0 for one of these coefficients implies that its associated covariate has no effect. A positive value means that an increase in the value of the associated covariate leads to an increase in survival time, that is, that larger values of the covariate are better. A negative coefficient means that an increase in the value of the associated covariate leads to lesser times, that is, that larger values of the covariate are worse. Note that this is the opposite of the situation for the regression coefficients in the proportional hazards model. But the difference between these models goes beyond this. Remember that in the proportional hazards model, you are modeling the effect of a covariate on the hazard function. In the accelerated failure time model, you are modeling the effect of a covariate on the survival times themselves.

Consider a covariate, *x,* which has the value 0 for the standard treatment and 1 for the experimental treatment. Suppose that in the model given by equation 1, its coefficient is 0.5. By equation 1, that means that the logarithm of the survival time is increased by 0.5 for the experimental treatment. Equivalently, the survival times for that treatment are exp(0.5) or about 1.65 times the survival times for the standard treatment. If the median survival time for the standard treatment is 3 years, then the median survival time for the experimental treatment is 3 times 1.65 or 4.95 years. Similar statements can be made for other percentiles. That is, the value of a covariate accelerates (or decelerates if the beta coefficient is negative) the time until a certain proportion of the mortality occurs. This provides the motivation for calling this the accelerated failure time model. By contrast, if the proportional hazards model produces an estimate of -0.5 for the coefficient of the treatment covariate, that means that the survival probabilities for the experimental treatment equal the corresponding probability for the standard treatment raised to the exp(-0.5) or about 0.61 power. If the median survival time for the standard treatment is 3 years, then the probability that a patient treated with the experimental treatment will survive at least 3 years is $0.5^{0.61}$ or about 66%.

3. PROC LIFEREG

PROC LIFEREG uses a syntax very much like that of PROC PHREG. After the PROC statement

```
proc lifereg;
```

you need a MODEL statement. This statement can take one of three forms. The first, which can be used if there is no left or interval censoring, is the same as that of PROC PHREG except for the optional specification of a distribution.

```
model timevar*censvar(censvals) = covariates / d = distribution;
```

Here *timevar* is the time variable, *censvar* is the variable that tells whether the time is right censored or not, *censvals* is a list of values of *censvar* that indicate that the time is right censored, and *covariates* is the list of covariates to be considered in the model. You specify the type of distribution for the time variable after the slash. The permissable choices are EXPONENTIAL, WEIBULL, GAMMA, LOGNORMAL, and LOGLOGISTIC. WIEBULL is the default. Later, some considerations that may help to make that choice are discussed. If you wish to allow for left and/or interval censoring, then the MODEL statement must take the form

```
model (timelo, timehi) = covariates / d = distribution;
```

Here *timelo* and *timehi* are time variables as described in section 1. If *timelo* is missing, then *timehi* is considered a left censored time. If *timehi* is missing, then *timelo* is considered a right censored time. If neither is missing and *timelo* < *timehi,* then the time is interval censored in the interval (*timelo, timehi*). If both are equal and not missing, then the time is uncensored at their common value.

There is a third form of MODEL statement syntax that is not generally used in survival analyses and is not discussed here. In both of the above forms, the covariates can be omitted. In that case, only the intercept, scale parameter, and, if gamma is chosen as the distribution for ε, a shape parameter, will be estimated.

PROC LIFEREG has no provision for specifying a method of entering or dropping covariates. You can, however, try several different models in the same invocation of the procedure by using several different MODEL statements. These models may differ in the distribution as well as the covariates used. This permits you to perform various significance tests "by hand." This process is demonstrated in the next example.

4. An Example of the Use of PROC LIFEREG

Let's reconsider the melanoma example discussed in the previous chapter. Patients with melanoma had their tumors removed surgically and were followed for relapse. Among the tumor characteristics that were studied for their effect on relapse time were the Clark and Breslow scores of the tumor. The following statements can be used to study the effect of these scores in models based on exponential, Weibull, and gamma distribution for the time to recurrence.

```
proc  lifetest;
    model dfstime*dfscens(0) = clark breslow / d = exponential;
    model dfstime*dfscens(0) = clark breslow;
    model dfstime*dfscens(0) = clark breslow / d = gamma;
    run;
```

The output is printed as Output 5.1.

Output 5.1

```
                         The SAS System

                      Lifereg  Procedure

Data Set           =WORK.MELANOMA
Dependent Variable=Log(DFSTIME)
Censoring Variable=DFSCENS
Censoring Value(s)=      0
Noncensored Values=   275  Right Censored Values=   1010
Left Censored Values=   0  Interval Censored Values=   0
Observations with Missing Values=  98
Observations with Zero or Negative Response=  13

Log Likelihood for EXPONENT -742.4698271    ❹
```

```
                        The SAS System

                     Lifereg   Procedure
                         ❷              ❸
Variable   DF    Estimate  Std Err  ChiSquare   Pr>Chi Label/Value
INTERCPT   1  6.49733516 0.326373   396.3168   0.0001 Intercept
CLARK      1  -0.3926619 0.098908   15.76055   0.0001 ❶
BRESLOW    1  -0.2067146 0.038011   29.57444   0.0001
SCALE      0            1         0                   Extreme value
    Lagrange Multiplier ChiSquare for Scale 32.45002 Pr>Chi is
                         0.0001.


                        The SAS System

                     Lifereg   Procedure


Data Set            =WORK.MELANOMA
Dependent Variable=Log(DFSTIME)
Censoring Variable=DFSCENS
Censoring Value(s)=      0
Noncensored Values=   275  Right Censored Values=    1010
Left Censored Values=   0  Interval Censored Values=    0
Observations with Missing Values=  98
Observations with Zero or Negative Response=  13


Log Likelihood for WEIBULL  -731.757061  ❹

                        The SAS System

                     Lifereg   Procedure
                         ❷              ❸
Variable   DF    Estimate  Std Err  ChiSquare   Pr>Chi Label/Value

INTERCPT   1   6.0917069 0.274405   492.8254   0.0001 Intercept
CLARK      1  -0.3415831 0.080442   18.03111   0.0001 ❶
BRESLOW    1  -0.1815029 0.030888   34.52837   0.0001
SCALE      1  0.81100079 0.034685                     Extreme value

                        The SAS System

                     Lifereg   Procedure


Data Set            =WORK.MELANOMA
Dependent Variable=Log(DFSTIME)
Censoring Variable=DFSCENS
Censoring Value(s)=      0
Noncensored Values=   275  Right Censored Values=    1010
Left Censored Values=   0  Interval Censored Values=    0
Observations with Missing Values=  98
Observations with Zero or Negative Response=  13


Log Likelihood for GAMMA -731.2938041  ❹
```

```
                        The SAS System

                     Lifereg  Procedure
                  ❷                   ❸
Variable   DF    Estimate  Std Err  ChiSquare  Pr>Chi Label/Value

INTERCPT   1  6.07093664  0.277994  476.9152   0.0001 Intercept
CLARK      1 -0.3429084   0.082103   17.44387  0.0001 ❶
BRESLOW    1 -0.1884148   0.033395   31.83285  0.0001
SCALE      1  0.88242566  0.082996                     Gamma scale p
SHAPE      1  0.83733927  0.160552                     Gamma shape p
```

Note the following features of Output 5.1:

❶   In all of the models, the effects of the BRESLOW and CLARK scores are highly significant.

❷   The fact that the coefficients of both are negative is consistent with what was seen in the proportional hazards model of Chapter 4. Higher values of these covariates are associated with shorter recurrence times. Specifically, a coefficient of -0.34 for the CLARK score implies that for each unit increase in this score, recurrence times are reduced by being multiplied by $\exp(-0.34) = 0.71$.

❸   Each Chi Square statistic is the square of the ratio of the estimate to its standard error. The p-value (Pr > Chi) is from a χ^2 distribution with 1 degree of freedom and is for a test that the associated parameter is 0. The CLARK and BRESLOW scores are significantly nonzero in all three models. These test statistics are not given for SCALE and SHAPE parameters. The SCALE parameter is forced to equal 1 in the EXPONENTIAL model. The SCALE parameter is estimated for the WEIBULL and GAMMA models, and the SHAPE parameter is estimated for the GAMMA model. In these cases, 0 is on the boundary of the the parameter's possible interval. The Chi Square test statistic described here does not provide a valid test in such cases.

❹   The log likelihood given for each model is the logarithm of the likelihood evaluated at the maximum likelihood estimators of the parameters. The larger it is, the more "likely" the sample under that model. Hence, the larger the log likelihood, the stronger the case is for that model. Note that because log likelihoods will be negative (being the logarithms of numbers between 0 and 1), larger log likelihoods have smaller absolute values.

5. Comparison of Models

The next question to be considered is how to tell which of two or more models is to be preferred. While larger maximum log likelihoods indicate a better model for the observed data, models with more parameters have, in general, larger log likelihoods. In fact, suppose that model A is a restriction of model B, perhaps by fixing one or more parameters at some value like 0 or 1. Then model B will almost certainly have a larger log likelihood than model A. To see why that is, suppose, for this example, that model B has two parameters, θ_1 and θ_2, and that they can be any real numbers and that θ_2 is restricted to be 0 in model A. When you find the maximum log likelihood for model B, you are finding the maximum value of a function over all possible pairs (θ_1, θ_2). However, when you maximize the log likelihood for model A, you are maximizing the same function over only those pairs for which θ_2 is 0. Unless the maximum likelihood estimator of θ_2 is 0, which is very unlikely, some (θ_1, θ_2) pair with $\theta_2 \neq 0$ will have a larger log likelihood than the log likelihood for any pair with $\theta_2 = 0$. A similar type of reasoning would work for any situation in which one model was a restriction of another. Because of this, you would not prefer model B to model A unless its log likelihood was sufficiently larger than that of model A, so that the excess was unlikely to be attributed to chance. Chapter 4, Section 11.1, "An Introduction to Likelihood-Based Estimation and Inference," tells us something about the distribution of the difference of two such log likelihoods. Here's the basic principle:

> Consider a model with m parameters and a null hypothesis that states that k of them have certain fixed values. Let L_m be the log likelihood maximized over all m parameters. Let L_{m-k} be the log likelihood maximized over the $m - k$ parameters not fixed by the null hypothesis, with the other k parameters having the values specified in the null hypothesis. Then, under the null hypothesis, $2(L_m - L_{m-k})$ has a χ^2 distribution with k degrees of freedom.

The above principle works equally well if the restriction of the null hypothesis states that certain regression coefficients have specified values, usually 0, or that one or more of the parameters of the baseline distribution have a specified value, usually 0 or 1.

Consider the three models for the melanoma data discussed previously. The Weibull distribution is a special case of the gamma distribution with the shape parameter equal to 1. Using the above notation, $L_m = L_3 = -731.2938041$ and $L_{m-k} = L_2 = -731.757061$ are the maximum log likelihoods for the gamma and Weibull models respectively. Start with the assumption of a gamma model, and test the restriction in which the shape parameter is 1, that is, that the data fit a Weibull distribution. Under the null hypothesis that the shape parameter is 1, $2(L_3 - L_2)$ has a χ^2 distribution with 1 degree of freedom. In this case $2(L_3 - L_2) = 0.92652$, which is not significant. In fact, the p-value is 0.34. You conclude that the data do not provide evidence that the shape parameter is not 1. Hence, you would not prefer the gamma model over the Weibull. Because the exponential distribution is a special case of the Weibull with the scale parameter equal to 1, this approach can be repeated to compare these distributions. Because L_1, the maximum log likelihood for the exponential model, is -742.4698271, $2(L_2 - L_1) = 21.42562$ and the data provide strong evidence ($p < .0001$) that the scale parameter is not 1, that is, that the data are not modeled by an exponential distribution. Note that the above discussion does not establish that tumor relapse time in this population follows a Weibull distribution. All that can be said is that in the heirarchy of exponential, Weibull, and gamma distributions, the Weibull is to be preferred. Later sections of this chapter discuss graphical methods of assessing the reasonableness of certain models.

6. Estimates of Quantiles and Survival Probabilities

PROC LIFEREG offers a rich set of additional options and features. Not all are discussed here. One useful feature is the ability to provide information about the estimated survival distribution defined by the model for specific covariate values. By using an OUTPUT statement, you can produce a data set that can provide survival function estimates in two ways. First, it can give the value of the cumulative distribution determined by the model for each patient, based on that patient's observed time and covariate values. Recall that the survival function is 1 minus the cumulative distribution function. Another way that PROC LIFEREG can provide information about the survival function for a patient with a specified set of covarariate values is to give the times associated with a set of quantiles of the cumulative distribution. The second approach is discussed below.

The OUTPUT statement goes after a MODEL statement and affects only the model that the preceeding MODEL statement defines. You may use OUTPUT statements with whichever MODEL statements you like. The syntax to accomplish what is described in the above paragraph is as follows:

```
output out = datasetname control = controlvar predicted = timevar
quantiles = list ;
```

Here, *datasetname* is the name of the output data set to be produced. It may be omitted. In that case, SAS names it using its DATA*n* convention. This is not recommended because it can be difficult to keep track of data sets named in this way. *list* is a list of probabilities for which you want the inverse of the cumulative distribution estimated. That is, if p is part of *list* then, for each patient, the time, t, for which $1 - \hat{S}(t) = p$ will be reported where $\hat{S}(t)$ is the estimated survival function determined by the model and the patient's covariate values. *list* can be of the form $p_1\,p_2\ldots p_k$ or p_1 to p_2 by *inc*. All values of p must be between 0 and 1. *timevar* is the name of the variable that will contain the time values for each quantile. The CONTROL = *controlvar* section is optional. It enables you to specify a variable, *controlvar*, in the data set used by PROC LIFEREG that controls the patients for whom these time values are estimated. If it is used, then the time values for each probability will be given only for those patients for whom *controlvar* = 1. If you want the quantiles for a specific set of covariate values, you can add to the DATA= data set an "artificial patient" with a missing time value, the desired covariate values, and a control variable that takes the value of 1. Because the time is missing, this "patient" will not affect the parameter estimates. However, the time for each probability in the quantile list will be produced. The output data set can, of course, be used with

SAS/GRAPH software to produce a graph of the estimated survival function. This is illustrated in the following example, which uses the melanoma data discussed previously.

```
data add;
   c = 1;
   clark = 2 ;
   breslow = .4;
   run;
data mel2;
   set melanoma add;
proc lifereg data = mel2;
   model dfstime*dfscens(0) = clark breslow;
   output out = weibull cdf = cdf predicted = months
   quantiles = 0.02 to 0.98 by .02
   control = c;

data dfs;
   set weibull;
   dfs_est = 1 - _prob_;
proc print;
   var  months dfs_est ;
   title 'Weibull Model with Clark = 2.0, Breslow = 0.4';
data;
   set dfs;
   if _n_ = 1 then do;
      dfs_est = 1.0 ;
      months = 0;
      output;
      end;
   output;
title1 h=2 f=swissb 'Figure 5.1';
title2 h=2 f=swissb 'Weibull Model for Melanoma DFS';
title3 h=2 f=swissb 'Clark = 2.0, Breslow = 0.4';
axis1 width=5 minor=none label=(h=3 f=swissb a=90 j=center
      'Pct DFS');
axis2 width=5 label=(h=3 f=swissb 'Months') value=(h=1.5 f=swissb);
symbol1 v=none l=1 i=spline ;
proc gplot;
   plot dfs_est*months;
run;
```

Note that a patient with the time variable missing, the control variable, C, defined to be 1, and covariate values of 2.0 and 0.4 for Clark and Breslow scores respectively, is added to the data set used by PROC LIFEREG. The variable C has a missing value for all other observations. The OUTPUT statement calls for calculating the times for which the cumulative distribution function (1 minus the survival function) is 0.02, 0.04, . . . , 0.96, 0.98. The output generated by PROC LIFEREG has already been given above. The output produced by invoking PROC PRINT to print the resultant data set (after subtracting the value of the probabilities from 1 to get DFS probabilities) is given as Output 5.2. The graph produced by SAS/GRAPH is Figure 5.1. Note that I=SPLINE was used to produce a smooth curve instead of the steps used in the Kaplan-Meier and proportional hazards estimates survival curve estimates. That is because, in this case, the graph is of a continuous function. In the other cases, the graphs were of functions whose values, by definition, were changed only at event times. Also notice that the graph is drawn well beyond the data that was used to estimate the parameters. No patients were observed for 500 months. Again, this is reasonable. Once we have estimates of the parameters, we can produce estimates of survival function values for all time values. Of course, survival function estimates for time values beyond those in the data set should be viewed skeptically.

Output 5.2

```
                        The SAS System
            Weibull Model with Clark = 2.0, Breslow = 0.4

                    OBS       MONTHS      DFS_EST

                     1         8.771        0.98
                     2        15.517        0.96
                     3        21.741        0.94
                     4        27.692        0.92
                     5        33.478        0.90
                     6        39.161        0.88
                     7        44.782        0.86
                     8        50.370        0.84
                     9        55.946        0.82
                    10        61.528        0.80
                    11        67.131        0.78
                    12        72.769        0.76
                    13        78.453        0.74
                    14        84.194        0.72
                    15        90.004        0.70
                    16        95.892        0.68
                    17       101.869        0.66
                    18       107.946        0.64
                    19       114.133        0.62
                    20       120.442        0.60
                    21       126.885        0.58
                    22       133.475        0.56
                    23       140.225        0.54
                    24       147.151        0.52
                    25       154.269        0.50
                    26       161.597        0.48
                    27       169.156        0.46
                    28       176.967        0.44
                    29       185.057        0.42
                    30       193.454        0.40
                    31       202.191        0.38
                    32       211.307        0.36
                    33       220.845        0.34
                    34       230.858        0.32
                    35       241.407        0.30
                    36       252.566        0.28
                    37       264.427        0.26
                    38       277.100        0.24
                    39       290.724        0.22
                    40       305.479        0.20
                    41       321.600        0.18
                    42       339.401        0.16
                    43       359.324        0.14
                    44       382.007        0.12
                    45       408.438        0.10
                    46       440.256        0.08
                    47       480.505        0.06
                    48       535.942        0.04
                    49       627.779        0.02
```

Figure 5.1

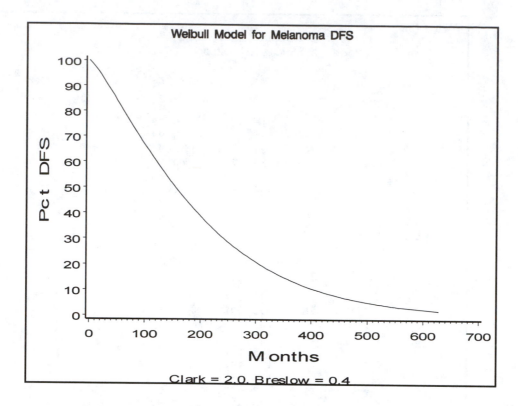

7. **The PROC LIFEREG Parameters and the "Standard" Parameters**

A little care is needed when relating the parameters of the accelerated failure time model of PROC LIFEREG to the usual parameterizations of the distributions used. The parameters estimated by the procedure are not the usual ones, but the relationships between the accelerated failure time model parameters and the model's usual parameters can be readily described. For example, suppose an exponential distribution is assumed and PROC LIFEREG is used to obtain estimates of β_0 and β', the intercept and the vector of regression coefficients for the covariate vector, $\mathbf{x}'$. Then, the hazard is a function of $\mathbf{x}$, which is written $\lambda(\mathbf{x})$. The survival function for a patient with covariate values given by $\mathbf{x}'$ is $S(t, \mathbf{x}) = \exp[-\lambda(\mathbf{x})t]$. It can then be shown that $\lambda(\mathbf{x}) = \exp-(\beta_0 + \beta'\mathbf{x}_1)]$. Thus $S(t, \mathbf{x}) = \exp\{-\exp[-(\beta_0 + \beta'\mathbf{x})]t\}$. Similarly, suppose you have assumed a Weibull model and used PROC LIFEREG to estimate β_0, and β' as above as well as σ, the scale parameter. The survival function for a patient with covariate vector $\mathbf{x}'$ can be written as $S(t, \mathbf{x}) = \exp(-\lambda(\mathbf{x})t^\gamma)$. Then $\lambda(\mathbf{x}) = \exp[-(\beta_0 + \beta'\mathbf{x})/\sigma]$ and $\gamma = 1/\sigma$.

8. The Macro PARAMEST

Although PROC LIFEREG can estimate the parameters of several of the more common survival distributions, it does not permit the user to specify any others. In particular, it does not permit consideration of models for which a nonzero proportion of patients are long-term survivors, or "cures." Such models, discussed previously in Chapter 1, have been the subject of a great deal of recent attention and interest by several authors (Goldman, 1984; Gamel et al. 1994; Cantor and Shuster, 1992).

The macro PARAMEST uses the IML procedure. It allows the user to specify any survival function and hazard function. These must be functions of a time variable named t and any number of parameters which must be named THETA[1], THETA[2], . . . , THETA[k]. Initial values as well as lower and upper bounds for the parameters may be provided. The optimization method usually works well with virtually any initial values. If a parameter is bounded, it is a good idea to include those bounds. This will keep the iteration from considering non-feasible parameter values that may create large log likelihoods. A module that calculates the log likelihood is used by the subroutine NLPTR, one of the nonlinear optimization subroutines that are included in PROC IML. This subroutine, and several other such subroutines, are described in the SAS manual *SAS/IML Software: Changes and Enhancements through Release 6.11*. You must be running Release 6.08 or later to use it. The subroutine NLPTR uses finite difference methods to estimate first and second derivatives of the log likelihood, if they are not provided as arguments. In order to make the macro PARAMEST as easy as possible to use, those arguments are not included. This adds considerably to the time needed to run the macro, but relieves the user of the need to provide first and second derivatives of the survival and hazard functions. If you often have the need to find MLE's for a particular model, you might want to modify the macro to include first, and perhaps second, derivatives as arguments to the subroutine. Another PROC IML function, NLLPFDD, which is also discussed in the previously mentioned manual, is used to estimate the matrix of second derivatives. This matrix is then inverted to obtain estimates of the covariance matrix of the parameter estimates. As an option, you may provide a data set that contains time and covariate values. In that case, estimates of the value of the survival probabilities for hypothetical patients with those times and covariate values are printed out as well. The macro PARAMEST uses the following arguments:

DATASET=

> This is the name of the data set containing the survival (and, optionally, covariate) data.

METHOD=

> This must be 1 or 2. It tells the macro which of two methods, as in PROC LIFEREG, are used to describe the survival data. If METHOD = 1, then the survival data are described by two time variables. If they are both nonmissing and the second is greater than the first, the time is taken to be interval censored in the interval they define. If the second is missing, the time is right censored at the first. If the first is missing, then the time is taken to be left censored at the second. Finally, if they are both nonmissing and are equal, then the time is complete at that common value. If METHOD=2, then only right censoring is permitted. Again two variables are needed to describe the survival data. The first is the observation time, and the second indicates whether that time is complete or right censored. The default value is 2.

T1=
T2=

These are the names of the time variables to be used. They describe survival time according to the method above. The defaults are T1 and T2.

COVS=

These are the names of the covariates. They should be listed with at least one space between them and no commas. The default is to have none.

CENSVAL=

This is used only with method 2 above. It is a row vector of the values that indicate a right censored observation. The time (first time variable) will be considered (right) censored if the value of the second time variable is one of those in this vector. The default is $\{0\}$.

HAZARD=

This is a formula for the hazard function. The parameters to be estimated must be named THETA[1], THETA[2], ... and so on. If you wish to consider covariates, they must be named X[1],X[2], ... and so on.

SURVIVAL=

This is a formula for the survival function. As for the hazard function, the parameters must be named THETA[1], THETA[2], ... and so on, and the covariates, if any, must be named X[1],X[2], ... and so on.

INIT=   This is a vector of initial values for the parameters, THETA[1], THETA[2], ... and so on. The macro will usually work well even if these are rather poor estimates.

UPPER=
LOWER=

These are vectors of upper and lower bounds, respectively, for the parameter, THETA[1], THETA[2], ... and so on. If there is no (upper or lower) bound for a parameter, that position in the vector should have a missing value. This can be used, for example, to indicate that a parameter can take on only positive values. In that case, the corresponding element of LOWER= should be a small positive value such 10^{-6}. The default is for all parameters to be unbounded.

ALPHA=

The macro PARAMEST produces $(1-ALPHA)*100\%$ confidence intervals for each of the parameters. The default value of ALPHA is 0.05.

PRED=

This is an optional data set that contains values of time and (if they are used) covariates at which survival probabilities and their standard errors are to be estimated. There should be no other variables in this data set. The first variable should be the time, and the others should be the same as those covariates in the VARS= argument above. The default is to have no such values. A word of caution is required here. In any SAS data set, the variables are ordered according to the order in which the compiler encountered them. If the data set PRED does not include any covariates, there will be no problem. If there are covariates as well as the time variable, then you must make sure that in creating the data set the compiler encounters the time variable first. For example, if there is a time variable, T, and two covariates, X1 and X2, and the data set is created with an INPUT statement, the INPUT statement must name the variable T first. That is, you can use

```
data;
    set pred;
    input t x1 x2;
    cards;
```

but not

```
data;
    set pred;
    input x1 x2 t;
    cards;
```

The macro can be called by using the template below.

```
%paramest(
          dataset =      /* The dataset to be used.
                            Default is _last_*/
          ,t1 =
          ,t2 =          /* Names of time variables. Defaults are
                            t1 and t2. */
          ,covs =        /* Names of the covariates. */
          ,method =      /* Method of specifying time.  Default is
                            2. */
          ,hazard =      /* Formula for the hazard function */
          ,survival =    /* Formula for the survival function */
          ,init =        /* Initial values for the parameters */
          ,alpha =       /* Used for confidence intervals for the
                            parameters.  Default value is 0.05.*/
          ,lower =       /* Lower bounds for parameters.  Default
                            is no lower bounds. */
          ,upper =       /* Upper bounds for parameters.  Default
                            is no upper bounds. */
          ,pred =        /* Data set containing time and,
                            optionally, covariate values for which
                            survival probabilities are to be
                            produced.  Default is none. */
          ,censval =     /* Value(s) that indicate censoring.
                            Default is {0} */
```

9. An Example of How to Use the Macro PARAMEST

As an example of how to use the macro PARAMEST, consider once again the data on disease-free survival of melanoma patients that was discussed above and analyzed with PROC LIFEREG. Again, the covariates Clark and Breslow will be used. This time the macro PARAMEST will be used to perform the same analyses. Although it would be possible for the parameters used by the macro to be the same INTERCEPT and SCALE parameters as in the previous example, it will be more instructive to use the usual parametrization of the Weibull distribution, $S(t) = \exp(\lambda t^\gamma)$. In using the macro, λ will be identified with THETA[1] and γ with THETA[2]. The macro PARAMEST allows you to model the effects of the covariates in a variety of ways. But for comparison with the results of PROC LIFEREG, assume an accelerated failure time model. From the discussion of section 7, it can be seen that that if X[1] and X[2] represent Clark and

Breslow, respectively, then the survival function incorporating these covariates can be written EXP($-$THETA[1]THETA[3]^{Clark}THETA[4]^{Breslow}T$^{THETA[2]}$). Letting β_0 be the intercept, β_1 and β_2 the coefficents of Clark and Breslow, and σ the scale parameter, the relationships between the parameters of this model and those of PROC LIFEREG are given by

THETA[1] = EXP($-\beta_0/\sigma$)
THETA[2] = $1/\gamma$
THETA[3] = EXP($-\beta_1/\sigma$)
THETA[4] = EXP($-\beta_2/\sigma$)

The following macro call estimates these parameters.

```
%paramest(
          t1=dfstime
         ,t2=dfscens
/* Names of time variables. Defaults are t1 and t2.   */
         ,covs=clark breslow
/* Names of the covariates */
         ,method=2
/* Method of specifying time.  Default is 2. */
         ,hazard=
theta[1]*theta[2]*theta[3]**x[1]*theta[4]**x[2]*t**(theta[2] - 1)
/* Formula for the hazard function */
         ,survival=
exp(-theta[1]*theta[3]**x[1]*theta[4]**x[2]*t**theta[2])
/* Formula for the survival function */
         ,init={1 1 1 1}
/* Initial values for the parameters */
              ,lower = {.0001 .0001 .0001 .0001}
 /* Lower bounds for parameters.  Default is no lower bounds. */
              ,upper = {10 10 10 10}
/* Upper bounds for parameters. Default is no upper bounds. */
)
```

The results of this call are given in Output 5.3.

Output 5.3

```
                    Successfull Convergence
                      MAXLL
                    -1601.163   Is Maximum Loglikelihood.

                         Parameter Estimate

        OBS      THETA      STDERR      LOWER       UPPER

         1      0.00066    0.00026     0.00015     0.00116
         2      1.18985    0.05120     1.08950     1.29021
         3      1.52837    0.15049     1.23341     1.82333
         4      1.24141    0.04713     1.14905     1.33378


                    Estimated Covariance Matrix

    Cov        theta1        theta2        theta3        theta4

  theta1    0.000000067   -.0000076    -0.00003     0.0000011
  theta2    -.000007560    0.0026218    0.000490    0.0002365
  theta3    -.000032041    0.0004895    0.022648    -.0028727
  theta4    0.000001133    0.0002365    -0.002873    0.0022209
```

Note that these estimates for THETA[1] – THETA[4] match those for the parameter estimates produced by PROC LIFEREG when the equations of section 9 are applied. The columns named LOWER and UPPER contain the bounds for 95% confidence intervals, since the default ALPHA= value of 0.05 was used.

The following example shows how to produce estimates of survival probabilities based on this model for a patient with a specified value for Clark and Breslow. Note that in creating the data set, PRED, the time variable T is the first to be encountered.

```
data pred;
    do t = 10 to 500 by 10;
        clark = 2.0;
        breslow = 0.4;
        output;
        end;
%paramest(
            dataset = melanoma
          ,t1 = dfstime, t2= dfscens
/* Names of time variables. Defaults are t1 and t2. */
          ,covs = clark breslow
/* Names of covariates. */
          ,hazard =
theta[1]*theta[2]*theta[3]**x[1]*theta[4]**x[2]*t**(theta[2] - 1)
/* Formula for the hazard function */
          ,survival =
exp(-theta[1]*theta[3]**x[1]*theta[4]**x[2]*t**theta[2])
/* Formula for the survival function */
          ,init = {1 1 1 1}
/* Initial values for the parameters */
          ,lower = {.0001 .0001 .0001 .0001}
/* Lower bounds for parameters.  Default is no lower bounds. */
          ,upper = {10 10 10 10}
/* Upper bounds for parameters. Default is no upper bounds. */
          ,pred = pred
);
run;
```

This time a data set, PRED, is specified. That data set has Clark = 2.0 and Breslow = 0.4 in each observation and T = 10, 20, . . . , 500. The additional results are in Output 5.4. You might wish to compare it to Output 5.2.

Output 5.4

		Estimated Survival Probabilities		
T	CLARK	BRESLOW	SURVIVAL	STDERR
10	2	0.4	0.97447	0.004417
20	2	0.4	0.94271	0.008857
30	2	0.4	0.90884	0.013287
40	2	0.4	0.87407	0.017655
50	2	0.4	0.83902	0.021915
60	2	0.4	0.80409	0.026023
70	2	0.4	0.76955	0.029945
80	2	0.4	0.73561	0.033655
90	2	0.4	0.70240	0.037134
100	2	0.4	0.67003	0.040365
110	2	0.4	0.63858	0.043341
120	2	0.4	0.60809	0.046056
130	2	0.4	0.57860	0.048507
140	2	0.4	0.55014	0.050698
150	2	0.4	0.52272	0.052630
160	2	0.4	0.49635	0.054311

170	2	0.4	0.47101	0.055747
180	2	0.4	0.44670	0.056947
190	2	0.4	0.42341	0.057921
200	2	0.4	0.40112	0.058679
210	2	0.4	0.37981	0.059233
220	2	0.4	0.35945	0.059594
230	2	0.4	0.34002	0.059775
240	2	0.4	0.32149	0.059786
250	2	0.4	0.30383	0.059640
260	2	0.4	0.28702	0.059348
270	2	0.4	0.27103	0.058922
280	2	0.4	0.25583	0.058374
290	2	0.4	0.24138	0.057713
300	2	0.4	0.22766	0.056952
310	2	0.4	0.21465	0.056099
320	2	0.4	0.20230	0.055165
330	2	0.4	0.19060	0.054160
340	2	0.4	0.17951	0.053091
350	2	0.4	0.16901	0.051967
360	2	0.4	0.15907	0.050796
370	2	0.4	0.14967	0.049586
380	2	0.4	0.14078	0.048344
390	2	0.4	0.13238	0.047075
400	2	0.4	0.12444	0.045787
410	2	0.4	0.11694	0.044484
420	2	0.4	0.10986	0.043172
430	2	0.4	0.10319	0.041856
440	2	0.4	0.09689	0.040539
450	2	0.4	0.09095	0.039227
460	2	0.4	0.08535	0.037922
470	2	0.4	0.08008	0.036628
480	2	0.4	0.07511	0.035348
490	2	0.4	0.07043	0.034084
500	2	0.4	0.06602	0.032839

10. An Example with a Positive Cure Rate

In the previous example, the macro PARAMEST was used to estimate the parameters of a Weibull survival distribution for a set of survival data that was previously analyzed using PROC LIFEREG. Although it was interesting to compare the two approaches, there would normally be little advantage of using this macro in this way. Indeed, the macro approach required a much greater amount of computer time. The real reason for presenting the macro PARAMEST is to enable you to perform analyses based on models not covered by PROC LIFEREG.

Consider the data set describing the survival of children with leukemia that was introduced in Chapter 2, section 9. Figure 2.3, a graph of the Kaplan-Meier survival curve, suggests that there are a nonzero proportion of "cures." In other words, the survival curve approaches a nonzero number as time increases. None of the functions allowed by PROC LIFEREG can have this property. Here are two ways of forming survival functions that have positive cure rates:

- Let $S(t) = \pi + (1 - \pi)S^*(t)$ where $0 < \pi < 1$ and $S^*(t)$ is any survival function that goes to 0 as t increases. Then π is the "cure rate" and $S^*(t)$ is the survival function for those not "cured." The mostly widely considered function of this type is formed by letting $S^*(t)$ be exponential. Thus $S(t) = \pi + (1 - \pi)\exp(-\lambda t)$. The hazard function is given by $h(t) = \lambda(1 - \pi)\exp(-\lambda t)/S(t)$.

- Let the function $h(t)$ be nonnegative (defined for all nonnegative values of t) and have the property that

$$\int_0^t h(u)\,du$$

approaches some number c as t increases without bound. It is seen in elementary calculus courses that this last property holds if and only if the series

$$\sum_{i=0}^{\infty} h(i)$$ converges. Then, the survival function

$S(t)$ defined by $S(t) = \exp[-\int_0^t h(u)\,du]$ approaches $\exp(-c)$, which is the

cure rate, as t increases without bound.

The most widely considered function of this type is formed by letting $h(t) = \alpha\exp(\beta t)$ where $\alpha > 0$. This hazard is initially (at $t = 0$) α and is changing exponentially at rate β.

This function is known as the Gompertz function. If $\beta < 0$ then

$$S(t) = \exp[-\int_0^t h(u)\,du]$$

which is $\exp\{-\alpha/\beta[\exp(\beta t) - 1]\}$ approaches $\exp(\alpha/\beta)$ as t increases without bound. The "cure rate" is given by $\exp(\alpha/\beta)$.

The following SAS statements use two macro calls to estimate the parameters of the two survival functions described above and to calculate estimated survival probabilities for $t = 1, 2, \ldots 10$ years. In both cases, initial values for the parameters were found by noting from the graph that the cure rate seems to be about 0.60 and that the two-year survival is about 0.70. These two values allow for an initial estimate of the parameters.

```
data pred;
   do t = 0 to 12;
   output;
   end;

title2 'Exponential with Cure Model';

%paramest(dataset =leuk
,hazard = (1 - theta[1])*theta[2]*exp(-theta[2]*t)/
          (theta[1] + (1 - theta[1])*exp(-theta[2]*t))
,t1 = time
,t2 = d
,method = 2
,survival = theta[1] + (1 - theta[1])*exp(-theta[2]*t)
,init={.6 .7}
,pred = pred
```

```
,lower = {.0001 .0001}
,upper = {.9999 .}
)

%paramest(
dataset =leuk
,hazard = theta[1]*exp(theta[2]*t)
,t1 = time
,t2 = d
,method = 2
,survival=exp(-(theta[1]/theta[2])*(exp(theta[2]*t)-1))
,init={.3 -.6}
,pred = pred
,lower = {.0001 .}
,upper = {. .}
)
```

The output is given in Output 5.5. The first part is for the exponential model. It estimates the "cure rate" to be about 0.61 and the constant hazard for the non-cures to be about 0.30/yr. These are the two values in the THETA column for that model. The second is for the Gompertz model. It estimates the initial hazard to be about 0.13/yr. and its exponential rate of change to be about −0.25/yr/yr. These are the two values in the THETA Gompertz model. The resultant estimated cure rate is about $\exp(-0.13/0.25) = 0.60$. Note that the two models predict almost indistinguishable survival probabilities and that these values are similar to those calculated by the Kaplan-Meier method in Chapter 2. In an article by Laska (1992), it is shown that the final Kaplan-Meier estimate is a reasonable nonparametric estimate for a cure rate. It is not surprising that different cure rate estimation methods yield similar results when applied to data sets with a lengthy follow-up period.

Output 5.5

```
                    Exponential with Cure Model

                     Successfull Convergence

                MAXLL
                -85.77513   Is Maximum Loglikelihood.

                        Parameter Estimates
        OBS      THETA      STDERR       LOWER        UPPER

          1     0.60707    0.068234     0.47333      0.74081
          2     0.30533    0.089005     0.13088      0.47977

                    Estimated Covariance Matrix

              Cov         theta1         theta2

            theta1       .0046559       .001791
            theta2       .0017915       .0079220

              Estimated Survival Probabilities

              T      SURVIVAL       STDERR
              0      1.00000      0.00000
              1      0.89661      0.026712
              2      0.82043      0.041427
              3      0.76429      0.049234
              4      0.72292      0.053344
              5      0.69244      0.055667
              6      0.66998      0.057247
              7      0.65343      0.058573
```

```
                   8      0.64123     0.059826
                   9      0.63224     0.061036
                  10      0.62562     0.062177
                  11      0.62074     0.063220
                  12      0.61714     0.064141


                      Gompertz Model
                  Successfull Convergence


                          MAXLL
                  -85.82645   Is Maximum Loglikelihood.


                     Parameter Estimates
        OBS       THETA       STDERR        LOWER         UPPER

         1      0.12690     0.039649      0.04919       0.20462
         2     -0.24865     0.086704     -0.41859      -0.07872


              Estimated Covariance Matrix

           Cov         theta1         theta2

         theta1      0.0015721     -.0025601
         theta2     -.0025601      0.0075176


              Estimated Survival Probabilities

            T      SURVIVAL       STDERR
            0      1.00000      0.000000
            1      0.89373      0.028403
            2      0.81875      0.042358
            3      0.76467      0.049221
            4      0.72499      0.052728
            5      0.69548      0.054781
            6      0.67330      0.056309
            7      0.65650      0.057722
            8      0.64368      0.059154
            9      0.63387      0.060619
           10      0.62631      0.062078
           11      0.62049      0.063487
           12      0.61598      0.064807
```

11. Comparison of Groups

In addition to providing a way of estimating parameters, the method of maximum likelihood also enables us to compare two or more groups. In Chapters 3 and 4, such comparisons focused only on whether one group was better than another with respect to survival. If you are willing to assume that two groups have the same type of survival function (for example, Weibull) with possibly different parameters, then it is easy to use the results of PROC LIFEREG or the macro PARAMEST to construct a test of the equivalence of the survival functions, that is, the equality of the parameter vectors. Tests can also be constructed to compare specific parameters or subsets of parameters.

11.1 An Omnibus Test

Consider two groups, 1 and 2, which are assumed to have the same type of survival distribution but with possibly different parameter vectors θ_1 and θ_2. The null hypothesis of equivalent survival distributions in these groups can be expressed as $\theta_1 = \theta_2$. The alternative is that $\theta_1 \neq \theta_2$. To construct a test statistic for this null hypothesis, you can run either PROC LIFEREG or the macro PARAMEST three times. In each case, note the value for the maximum loglikelihood. The first time use only those observations in group 1. The second time use only those observations in group 2. Call these maximum log likelihoods LL_1 and LL_2 respectively. The third time use all of the observations. Call the resultant maximum log likelihood LL_0. Now the maximum log likelihood for the combined sample under the alternative is $LL_1 + LL_2$. This follows from the fact that the likelihood for the combined sample is the product of the separate likelihoods, hence the maximum log likelihood for the combined sample is the sum of the respective log likelihoods. LL_0 is the maximum log likelihood under the the null hypothesis. Using the principle for likelihood ratio tests stated at the end of Chapter 4, under the null hypothesis, the statistic $2(LL_1 + LL_2 - LL_0)$ has a χ^2 distribution with degrees of freedom equal to the number of parameters in the model. The null hypothesis is, therefore, rejected if that statistic exceeds the critical value associated with the chosen significance level for that χ^2 distribution.

As an example, turn once again to the melanoma data that were previously analyzed. This time, define two groups according to Clark score, which takes on the values of 1, 2, 3, and 4. Group 1 will consist of those with a Clark score of 4. Group 2 will be all others. The following statements enable you to test the null hypothesis that, in a Weibull model, the intercept and scale parameters in these two groups are the same against the alternative that at least one of them differs.

```
data melanoma;
   set melanoma;
   group=2-(clark=4);
proc sort;
   by group;
proc lifereg;
   model dfstime*dfscens(0) = ;
   by group;
   title 'Individual Groups';
run;
proc lifereg;
   model dfstime*dfscens(0) =;
   title 'Combined Sample';
run;
```

The output is in Output 5.6.

Output 5.6

```
                          Individual Groups

----------------------------- GROUP=1-------------------
                        Lifereg    Procedure

Data Set           =WORK.MELANOMA
Dependent Variable=Log(DFSTIME)
Censoring Variable=DFSCENS
Censoring Value(s)=    0
Noncensored Values=   172   Right Censored Values=    432
Left Censored Values=   0   Interval Censored Values=   0
Log Likelihood for WEIBULL -453.4687154
```

```
                            Individual Groups


---------------------------- GROUP=1 ------------------

                          Lifereg   Procedure

Variable  DF   Estimate  Std Err ChiSquare  Pr>Chi Label/Value

INTERCPT   1 4.34595117 0.079369  2998.234   0.0001 Intercept
SCALE      1 0.91660179 0.051987                    Extreme value scale
                            Individual Groups


---------------------------- GROUP=2 ------------------

                          Lifereg   Procedure

Data Set          =WORK.MELANOMA
Dependent Variable=Log(DFSTIME)
Censoring Variable=DFSCENS
Censoring Value(s)=     0
Noncensored Values=   113  Right Censored Values=     577
Left Censored Values=   0  Interval Censored Values=   0


Log Likelihood for WEIBULL -321.0223407

                            Individual Groups

---------------------------- GROUP=2 --------------------
                          Lifereg   Procedure

Variable  DF   Estimate  Std Err ChiSquare  Pr>Chi Label/Value

INTERCPT   1 4.89447835 0.092569  2795.663   0.0001 Intercept
SCALE      1 0.77839429 0.051887                    Extreme value scale
                            Combined Sample

                          Lifereg   Procedure

Data Set          =WORK.MELANOMA
Dependent Variable=Log(DFSTIME)
Censoring Variable=DFSCENS
Censoring Value(s)=     0
Noncensored Values=   285  Right Censored Values=    1009
Left Censored Values=   0  Interval Censored Values=   0


Log Likelihood for WEIBULL -797.9950515

                            Combined Sample

                          Lifereg   Procedure

Variable  DF   Estimate  Std Err ChiSquare  Pr>Chi Label/Value

INTERCPT   1 4.66573806 0.063277  5436.941   0.0001 Intercept
SCALE      1 0.88509116 0.038424                    Extreme value scale
```

For the results above, you can calculate that $2(LL_1 + LL_2 - LL_0)$ exceeds 23, which is highly significant. The critical value for the χ^2 distribution with 2 degrees of freedom for significance level 0.001 is 13.8. Thus, these results offer strong evidence that the distributions for those with Clark score of 4.0 and those with Clark score less than 4.0 are different.

11.2 Individual Parameters

Results such as those seen in 11.1 can also provide insight into whether two groups differ in the values of individual parameters. In general, the estimates are approximately normally distributed with the standard deviations equal to the standard errors in the output. Furthermore, under the null hypotheses that the parameters they estimate are equal, they have the same expected value, namely that common parameter value. Thus, their difference under the null hypothesis has a normal distribution with mean zero and variance equal to the sum of the variances of the estimates. If the parameter estimates in the two goups are denoted $\hat{\theta}_1$ and $\hat{\theta}_2$ and their standard errors are s_1 and s_2, then, under the null hypothesis, the statistic $(\hat{\theta}_1 - \hat{\theta}_2) / \sqrt{s_1 + s_2}$ has a standard normal distribution. The null hypothesis is rejected for values that exceed, in absolute value, the critical value of the standard normal distribution for the desired significance level. For the groups in the above example, that statistic has a value of -4.50 for the intercept and 1.88 for the scale parameter. Thus, the evidence is quite strong that the two groups determined by Clark score differ in their intercept ($p < 0.001$). For the scale parameter, the evidence is marginal ($p = 0.06$).

12. One-Sample Tests of Parameters

The theory for maximum likelihood provides two ways to test null hypotheses of the form H_0: $\theta = \theta_0$ where θ is one of the parameters that characterize a survival distribution and θ_0 is a particular value. First of all, letting s be the standard error of the parameter estimate, $\hat{\theta}$, you can compare $(\hat{\theta} - \theta_0)/s$ to a critical value of a standard normal distribution. You reject the null hypothesis if the absolute value of $(\hat{\theta} - \theta_0)/s$ exceeds that critical value. Another approach is to use PROC LIFEREG or the macro PARAMEST twice. The first time, you want to calculate the MLE's of all of the distribution's parameters and the maximum log likelihood at those MLE's. The second time, you want to fix the value of θ, the parameter of interest, at its hypothesized value and calculate the remaining MLE's and the resultant maximum log likelihood. Note that the SCALE= and SHAPE= options in PROC LIFEREG enable you to restrict these values. The first of these maximum log likelihoods is the maximum log likelihood under the alternative that θ doesn't equal θ_0. Call it LL_A. The second is the maximum log likelihood under the alternative that θ equals θ_0. Call it LL_0. Then $2(LL_A - LL_0)$ has, under the null hypothesis, a χ^2 distribution with 1 degree of freedom. Reject the null hypothesis if that statistic exceeds the critical value for this distribution.

For an example, consider the leukemia data set discussed previously in this chapter. Suppose that you would expect, based on previous experience, to have a 50% cure rate for these patients if they had been given standard therapy. Do these data offer evidence that the therapy used in this study has a cure rate that differs from 50% ? Using the survival function $S(t) = \pi + (1 - \pi)\exp(-\lambda t)$, the results of section 10 show an estimated "cure rate" of 0.607 with a standard error of 0.068. The first test statistic discussed above is then $(0.607 - 0.500)/0.068 = 1.569$ which is not statistically significant ($p = 0.117$). Of course, this also follows from the fact that 0.500 is in the 95% confidence interval for this parameter. For a second approach, you can redo the invocation of the macro PARAMEST with THETA[1] fixed at 0.5 and compare the maximum log likelihood to that obtained without that restriction. That is, take $S(t) = 0.5 + 0.5\exp(-\lambda t)$ and $h(t) = 0.5\lambda\exp(-\lambda t)/[0.5 + 0.5\exp(-\lambda t)]$. The macro can be called by

```
%paramest(
          dataset =leuk
          ,hazard =
           .5*theta[1]*exp(-theta[1]*t)/(.5 +.5*exp(-theta[1]*t))
          ,t1 = time
          ,t2 = d
          ,method = 2
          ,survival = .5 +.5*exp(-theta[1]*t)
          ,init={.7}
          ,pred = pred
          ,lower = {.0001}
          ,upper = {.}
    )
```

The maximum log likelihood for this model is -86.81925. In section 5.10, it was seen that the maximum log likelihood for the unrestricted model was -85.77513. The second test statistic of the previous paragraph has the value $2[-85.77513 - (-86.81925)]$ $= 2.08824$. Referring to a χ^2 distribution with 1 degree of freedom, the p value is 0.148. This is similar to the result using the first method.

13. The Effects of Covariates on Parameters

In section 5.9, you saw how you could use the PARAMEST macro to evaluate the effect of covariates on the two parameters of the Weibull survival distribution. Let's look at this issue a bit more closely. Suppose there are k covariates, $x_1, x_2, \ldots, x_k$, being studied for their association with survival. Then, each of the parameters of a survival function could conceivably be affected by some or all of them. You might express a parameter, θ, as a linear function of these covariates, say $\beta_0 + \beta_1 x_1 + \ldots + \beta_k x_k$. Note that β_0 is then the baseline value of the parameter, that is, the value of the parameter when $x_1 = x_2 = \ldots = x_k = 0$. But this linear function can take on all real values, so this would not be a good way to express a parameter that had a more limited set of permissable values. If a parameter can take on only positive values, a better approach to expressing it as a function of the covariates might be to write it as $\exp(\beta_0 + \beta_1 x_1 + \ldots + \beta_k x_k)$. In this case, the baseline value is $\exp(\beta_0)$. If the parameter can take on only values between 0 and 1, as with a cure rate, then you might express it as $[1 + \exp(\beta_0 + \beta_1 x_1 + \ldots + \beta_k x_k)]^{-1}$. Then the baseline value becomes $[1 + \exp(\beta_0)]^{-1}$. Of course, different parameters being expressed as functions of the covariates will require distinct coefficients. A fairly large number of parameters may be needed to express a survival function in this way. If there are k covariates and p original parameters in the model, then a total of $p(k+1)$ parameters will be needed. We are fortunate to have powerful computers and software to perform matrix operations on matrices of this size.

A particularly interesting situation arises with a model for survival of the form $S(t) = \pi + (1 - \pi)S^*(t)$ where $S^*(t)$ is a survival function that gives survival probabilities for those not cured and where π is the cure rate. Suppose that $S^*(t)$ is determined by some parameter, θ. For simplicity, only one such parameter is considered here, although the extension to more than one will be obvious. Then, presumably, both π and θ could be affected by the values of a covariate, x. Again only one covariate will be considered. You might be interested in how x affects both the cure rate and the survival of the non-cures.

As an example, consider once again the leukemia data discussed in Chapters 2 and 3. You saw in Chapter 3 that two treatment groups did not differ significantly by the log rank test. Because both groups seem to have nonzero cure rates, you might want to assess the effect of treatment on the cure rate and the survival of those who are not cured. If survival is modeled by the exponential model with cure, then the survival and hazard functions become

$$S(t, x) = \frac{1}{1 + \exp(\theta_1 + \theta_2 x)} + $$

$$\frac{\exp(\theta_1 + \theta_2 x)}{1 + \exp(\theta_1 + \theta_2 x)} \exp[-\exp(\theta_3 + \theta_4 x)t]$$

and

$$h(t, x) = -\frac{S'(t, x)}{S(t, x)} \tag{2}$$

where x is 0 or 1 depending on the treatment group and

$$S'(t, x) = \frac{\exp(\theta_3 + \theta_4 x)\exp(\theta_1 + \theta_2 x)\exp[-\exp(\theta_3 + \theta_4 x)t]}{1 + \exp(\theta_1 + \theta_2 x)}$$

The following SAS statements estimate the four parameters above.

```
%paramest(dataset=leuk
           ,hazard=
exp(theta[3]+theta[4]*x[1])*(1-(1+exp(theta[1]+theta[2]*x[1]))**
(-1))*exp(-exp(theta[3]+theta[4]*x[1])*t)/
((1+exp(theta[1]+theta[2]*x[1]))**(-1)
+(1-(1+exp(theta[1]+theta[2]*x[1]))**(-1))*
exp(-exp(theta[3]+theta[4]*x[1])*t))
           ,t1=years
           ,t2=cens
           ,covs=group
           ,method=2
           ,survival=
(1+exp(theta[1]+theta[2]*x[1]))**(-1)
 +(1-(1+exp(theta[1]+theta[2]*x[1]))**(-1))*
exp(-exp(theta[3]+theta[4]*x[1])*t)
           ,init={0 0 .3 0}
)
```

The results are printed as Output 5.7.

Output 5.7

```
                    Successfull Convergence


                  MAXLL
              -182.0274   Is Maximum Loglikelihood.

                    Parameter Estimates

       OBS       THETA       STDERR       LOWER        UPPER

        1      -0.43501     0.28592     -0.99540      0.12538
        2       0.36080     0.41161     -0.44593      1.16754
        3      -1.18638     0.29140     -1.75751     -0.61524
        4      -0.11637     0.40314     -0.90651      0.67376

                 Estimated Covariance Matrix

    Cov          theta1       theta2        theta3       theta4

   theta1      0.081749    -0.08169     -0.024545      0.02450
   theta2     -0.081694     0.16942      0.024497     -0.05396
   theta3     -0.024545     0.02450      0.084915     -0.08486
   theta4      0.024501    -0.05396     -0.084864      0.16252
```

The second and fourth THETA values measure the effect of treatment on the cure rate and the hazard among the non-cures respectively. Note that neither are significant at the 0.05 significance level. This is seen by the fact that both 95% confidence intervals contain 0. Alternatively, you could refer the ratio THETA/STDERR to the standard normal distribution. The estimated cure rates are $1/[1 + \exp(-.43501)] = 0.607$ for group 0 and 0.519 for group 1. The corresponding hazard estimates are $\exp(-1.18638) = 0.305$ and 0.272.

Take a moment to compare the kind of information learned from this example to that which the log rank test can tell you. The log rank test only provides insight concerning the superiority of one group over the other. That insight comes from considering the relationship of the number of deaths in each group to the numbers that would have been expected if the groups had equivalent survivorship. The current approach is far more informative. It enables you to compare groups with respect to the proportion cured as well as the survival times of those not cured. Although it didn't happen in this example, it is quite possible for groups to not differ significantly by the log rank test, but for one to have a significantly higher cure rate. Of course, there is a price to pay for this more informative analysis – the parametric assumption. If the groups' true survival distributions are not given, at least approximately, by a function of the assumed form, the results will not be valid. Section 15 addresses this problem.

14. Complex Expressions for the Survival and Hazard Functions

One problem with the PARAMEST macro is that the expressions used with SURVIVAL= and HAZARD= can get quite complicated, as seen in the previous example. When that happens, it may be difficult to type them correctly. Here's a suggestion that you may find helpful. When a parameter is a function of covariates, first type the survival and hazard functions without considering the covariates. Then use "search and replace" to replace the parameters with the appropriate function of the covariates. In the example above, you might first type

```
survival=pi+(1-pi)*exp(-lambda*t)
```

Then use "search and replace" to replace PI by

```
1/(1+exp(theta[1]+theta[2]*x))
```

and to replace LAMBDA by

```
exp(theta[3]+theta[4]*x)
```

15. Graphical Checks for Certain Survival Distributions

Of course, all of the above is contingent upon the fact that the sample being analyzed comes from a population having a survival distribution of the type chosen. While such analyses can, as has been seen, be more informative than those done by the nonparametric or semiparametric methods of Chapters 2, 3, and 4, they are invalid if the population survival distribution is not, at least approximately, of the type chosen. There are, unfortunately, no methods for deciding whether or not a given type of distribution fits a set of survival data. The best we can do is to note that, for a certain type of survival functions, a simple relationship (such as linear) exists between some function of the survival function and some function of time. By plotting the graph of that relationship using Kaplan-Meier estimates of the survival function, and by noting whether or not it appears to be linear, you can determine whether or not a certain model is reasonable. Furthermore, the slope and intercept of the line can provide information about the parameters that can help determine initial values. The details of this approach, for several common models, is discussed in the following subsections.

15.1 The Exponential and Weibull Distributions

Consider a Weibull survival function, that is $S(t) = \exp(\lambda t^\gamma)$. Then, it is not hard to see that $\log_e[-\log_e(S(t)] = \log_e(\lambda) + \gamma \log_e(t)$. Thus if you obtain the Kaplan-Meier estimates, $\hat{S}(t)$, of $S(t)$, and plot a graph of $\log_e[-\log_e(\hat{S}(t)]$ versus $\log_e(t)$, that graph should be roughly linear if the data come from a Weibull distribution. The slope would then be γ. If that slope is about 1 then this indicates that $\gamma = 1$ and an exponential model is reasonable. Because $\log_e(\lambda)$ is the intercept, applying the exponential function to the intercept provides an initial estimate of λ. If you want a graphical check of exponentiality, you can use the fact that, if $S(t) = e^{-\lambda t}$, then $-\log_e[S(t)] = \lambda t$. Thus, you can consider the graph of $-\log_e[\hat{S}(t)]$ versus t. For exponential survival functions, this should be linear and go through the origin. The slope provides an initial estimate of λ. PROC LIFETEST provides the capability of producing these graphs. Simply include PLOTS = (LLS), PLOTS = (LS), or PLOTS = (LS, LLS) in the PROC statement for the graph of $\log_e\{-\log_e[S(t)]\}$ versus $\log_e(t)$, $\log_e[S(t)]$ versus t, or both.

15.2 The Lognormal Distribution

This distribution is given by $S(t) = \Phi\{[\log_e(t) - \mu]/\sigma\}$ where $\Phi(x)$ is the standard normal cumulative distribution function. It follows that $[\log_e(t) - \mu]/\sigma = \Phi^{-1}[S(t)]$. Again, letting $\hat{S}(t)$ be the Kaplan-Meier estimates of $S(t)$, you might consider the graph of $\log_e(t)$ versus $\Phi^{-1}[\hat{S}(t)]$. This can be done easily in SAS because SAS provides the inverse of the standard normal cumulative distribution as the PROBIT function. A lognormal distribution is indicated if that graph is approximately linear. Furthermore, the reciprocal of the slope will approximate σ. That value for σ multiplied by the negative of the intercept will approximate μ.

15.3 The Exponential Model with "Cure"

This survival distribution is given by $S(t) = \pi + (1 - \pi)\exp(-\lambda t)$. It follows that $-\log_e\{[S(t) - \pi]/(1 - \pi)\} = \lambda t$. You can plot the graphs of $-\log_e\{[\hat{S}(t) - \pi]/(1 - \pi)\}$ versus t for several values of π, where $\hat{S}(t)$ is the Kaplan-Meier estimate of $S(t)$. If one of them looks like a straight line through the origin, that indicates a model of this type. The value of π for this graph is an initial estimate of π, and the slope is an initial estimate of λ.

15.4 The Gompertz Model

The Gompertz survival curve has survival function $S(t) = \exp\{(-\alpha/\beta)[exp(\beta t) - 1]\}$. It will be convenient to rewrite it as $\pi^{1 - exp(\beta t)}$ where $\pi = \exp(\alpha/\beta)$. Recall that π is the cure rate if $\beta < 0$. It follows that $\log_e\{1 - \log_e[S(t)]/\log_e(\pi)\} = \beta t$. Letting $\hat{S}(t)$ be the Kaplan-Meier estimate of $S(t)$, you can plot the graphs of $\log_e\{1 - \log_e[\hat{S}(t)]/\log_e(\pi)\}$ versus t for several values of π. If one of them appears to be a straight line through the origin, that indicates that a Gompertz model is reasonable. The value of π for that graph is an initial estimate of the cure rate, or $\exp(\alpha/\beta)$. The slope of that line is an initial estimate of β.

16. A Macro for Fitting Parametric Models to Survival Data

The macro CHEKDIST allows you to perform on a data set the graphical checks described in section 15. To use it, you must provide information about the data set that contains the survival data and the model, chosen from those described above, that you wish to fit. For the Gompertz model or the exponential model with cure, you also need to provide the value (or values) of π which you would like to check. Those values are specified in list format. Some examples are

```
pi = 0.5
pi = 0.2 to 0.8 by 0.2
```

Because the macro processor interprets a comma as an indication that the parameter specification has ended, you cannot use an expression like

```
pi = 0.2, 0.3, 0.4
```

To invoke this macro, you can use the following template:

```
%chekdist(
            data =           /* The name of the dataset to be used.
                                Default is _last_ */
            ,time =          /* The name of the time variable   */
            ,cens =          /* The name of the censoring variable */
            ,censvals =      /* Values of the censoring variable that
                                indicate a censored observation.
                                Default is 0 */
            ,model =         /* Model to be fit.  Choices are exp,
                                weibull, lognorm, expcure, and gomp */
            ,pi =            /* Value(s) for the cure rate */
)
```

As examples, consider the two invocations of the macro CHEKDIST given below. The first checks on the fit of a Weibull model to a data set of survival data. The second checks on the fit of an exponential model with cure to another data set. Cure rates of 0.3, 0.4, 0.5, 0.6, and 0.7 are considered. In both data sets, the time variable is t and the censoring variable is CENS. The only censoring value is 0, which is the default. Both data sets were artificially created to have the distribution for which they are being checked. The data set DATA1 is simulated from a Weibull model with $\lambda = 0.33$ and $\gamma = 0.64$. The data set DATA2 is simulated from an exponential with cure model with $\lambda = 0.23$ and $\pi = 0.4$. The results are seen in Figures 5.2 and 5.3. Note that the graph in Figure 5.2 is nearly linear. This would support the contention that the underlying data was sampled from a Weibull distribution. The apparent departure from linearity seen in the far left part of this curve in due to one very early death in the simulated data set. Furthermore, the vertical coordinate associated with $\log_e(t) = 0$ is about -1.0. This would suggest a value for λ of about $\exp(-1.0) = 0.37$. The slope of the line appears to be about 0.6, suggesting that value for γ. Both values are close to those of the population sampled. In Figure 5.3, the graph for $\pi = 0.4$ is nearly linear. This indicates that a model with about 40% surviving and exponential survival for the non-cures is reasonable. The slope for the graph with $\pi = 0.4$ appears to be about -0.15, suggesting a value for λ of about 0.15.

```
%chekdist(
        data=data1    /* The name of the dataset to be used.
                         Default is _last_ */
        ,time=t       /* The name of the time variable  */
        ,cens=cens    /* The name of the censoring variable */
        ,model=weibull/* Model to be fit.  Choices are exp,
                         weibull, lognorm, expcure, and gomp */
)
title 'Check of Weibull Fit';


%chekdist(
        data=data2    /* The name of the dataset to be used.
                         Default is _last_ */
        ,time=t       /* The name of the time variable  */
        ,cens=cens    /* The name of the censoring variable */
        ,model=expcure /* Model to be fit.  Choices are exp,
                         weibull, lognorm, expcure, and gomp */
        ,pi = .3 to .7 by .1  /* Value(s) for the cure rate */
)
title 'Check of Exponenential with Cure Fit';
```

Figure 5.2

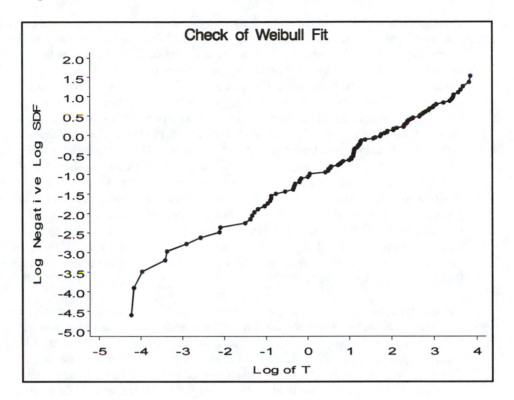

Figure 5.3

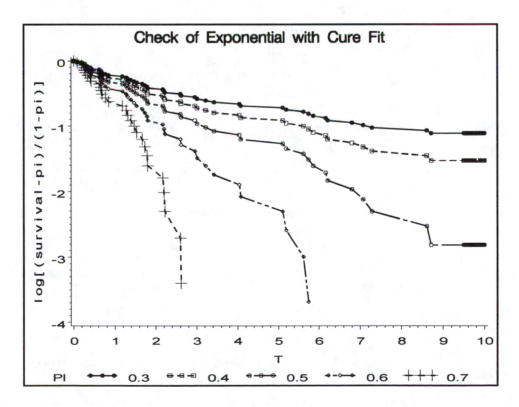

17. Other Estimates of Interest

If you assume a model for survival that implies that some patients are cured, then the cure rate is, of course, a critical parameter to estimate. This can be thought of as the probability that a patient entering the study will *not* die from the disease under consideration. Now suppose that probability for a given patient (perhaps based on covariate values) is π. If that patient is alive some time later, then it is reasonable to assume that the patient's chances of being a cure have been increased. Many investigators simply declare a patient cured when a certain survival time is achieved. Such a declaration is generally based on experience that indicates that patients who survive for that amount of time do not die of the disease. The methods discussed in this chapter allow an alternative approach to this question. It is not hard to show that the probability that a patient is cured, conditioned on having survived to time t, is given by $\pi/S(t)$. Replacing $S(t)$ and π with their estimates produces the estimated conditional probability. For example, consider a leukemia patient in the cohort whose survival is modeled above. Using the Gompertz model, that patient has, upon beginning the study, an estimated probability of about 0.60 of not succumbing to the disease. If this patient survives for three years, his or her probability of never dying from the disease is now 0.600/0.765, or about 0.784.

Another type of estimate that may be of interest is the survival function for those not cured. For a cohort with survival function $S(t)$ that approaches π as t increases, that function is given by $[S(t) - \pi]/(1 - \pi)$. Again, replacement of $S(t)$ and π with their estimates produces the estimated survival function for the non-cures. For example, applying the Gompertz model to the leukemia data, you could estimate that a patient not cured will have a probability of $(0.765 - 0.600)/(1 - 0.600) = 0.412$ of surviving for more than three years.

18. Complete Macros

18.1 The Macro PARAMEST

```
%macro paramest(dataset = _last_, t1=t1, t2=t2, covs=none,
                       method = 2,
            hazard =     , survival =  ,init= , alpha = 0.05,
            lower = {. . . . . . . . . .},
            upper = {. . . . . . . . . .},
            pred = x, censval = {0});

/*Remove Observations with Time Values That Are Not Permissable*/

data checked;
      set &dataset;
      if &method=1 and ((&t1 = . and &t2 = .) or &t1 > &t2
            or . < &t1 < 0 or . < &t2 < 0) then delete;
      if &method=2 and (&t1 < 0 or &t2 = . ) then delete;

/* to get rid of previous datasets */

data survival;
      set _null_;
data x;
      set _null_;

proc iml;
b = &upper;
      a = &lower;
      con = a//b;
      use checked;
      %if &covs = none %then
            %str(read all var {&t1 &t2} into vars;);
      %else %str(read all var {&t1 &t2 &covs} into vars;);
      nvars = ncol(vars);
```

```
              ncovs = nvars - 2;
              nobs = nrow(vars);
              times = vars[, 1:2];

/*  convert to method 1 for time and censoring data */

if &method = 2 then do i=1 to nobs;
   if sum((times[i,2] = &censval)) >0 then times[i,2] = .;
   else times[i,2] = times[i,1];
   end;

/* module to calculate log likelihood   */

              start loglik(theta) global (times,vars,nobs,nvars);
              LL=0;
              do i=1 to nobs;
      /*  get covariates  */

                  if nvars > 2 then x = vars[i,3:nvars];

      /*  right censored time */

                  if (times[i,1] ^= .) & (times[i,2] = . ) then do;
              t = times[i,1];
              LL = LL + log(&survival);
              end;

      /* left censored time */

        if (times[i,1] = .) & (times[i,2] ^= .) then do;
            t = times[i,2];
            LL = LL + log(1 - (&survival));
            end;

      /* interval censored time */

              if (times[i,1] ^= .) & (times[i,2] > times[i,1]) then do;
                  t = times[i,1];
              temp = &survival ;
              t = times[i,2];
              y = temp - (&survival) ;
              LL = LL + log(y);
              end;

      /* uncensored time */

              if times[i,1] = times[i,2] then do;
                  t=times[i,1];
                  LL = LL + log(&hazard) + log(&survival);
                  end;
          end;
          return(LL);
          finish loglik;
          theta0= &init`;
          nparams = ncol(&init);
          con = con[, 1:nparams];
          optn = {1 0};

/*  call optimization function */

          call nlptr(rc,thetares,"loglik",theta0,optn,con,,,,,);
          thetaopt=thetares`;
          maxll=loglik(thetaopt);
```

```
/*  rc is return code  - negative means failed to converge  */

        if rc < 0 then
        print "Iteration failed to converge.  Estimates are
        unreliable.";
        if rc > 0 then do;
                print "Successfull Convergence";
                print maxll " Is Maximum Loglikelihood.";
                end;

/* module to calculate first derivs (deriv) and second derivs (h)*/

        call nlpfdd(LL,deriv,h,"loglik", thetaopt);

/* get covariance matrix and standard errors of estimates */

        cov = -inv(h);
        setheta=sqrt(vecdiag(cov));
        theta=thetaopt;
        use &pred;
        read all var _all_ into values;
        n = nrow(values);
        survival = j(1,n,0);
        sesurv = j(1,n,0);
        covplus1 = ncovs + 1;

/* calculate survival function for t and covariates in pred
dataset, as well as statndard error using delta method */

        do i = 1 to n;
                if ncovs > 0 then x = values[i,2:covplus1];
                t = values[i,1];
                start surv(theta) global (i, t, x);
                surv = &survival;
                return(surv);
                finish surv;
                call nlpfdd(s,deriv,hess,"surv", theta);
                survival[i] = s;
                sesurv[i] = sqrt(deriv*cov*deriv`);
                end;
        survival = survival`;
        sesurv = sesurv`;
        create thetas from theta[colname = 'theta'];
        append from theta;
        create setheta from setheta[colname = 'stderr'];
        append from setheta;
        create cov from cov;
        append from cov;
        create survival from survival[colname = 'survival'];
        append from survival;
        create sesurv from sesurv[colname = 'stderr'];
        append from sesurv;
data thetas;
        merge thetas setheta;
        c = probit(1 - &alpha/2);

/*  (1 - alpha)100% CI */

        lower = theta - stderr*c;
        upper = theta + stderr*c;
proc print data = thetas;
        var theta stderr lower upper;
        title 'Parameter Estimates';
run;
proc means noprint n data = cov;
    var col1;
    output out = out n = nparams;
run;
data;
        set out;
        call symput('n', nparams);
run;
```

```
data names;
%do i = 1 %to &n;
        name = "theta&i";
        output;
        %end;
run;
data cov;
merge names cov;
proc print data= cov noobs label ;
%do i = 1 %to &n;
        label col&i = "theta&i";
        %end;
        label name = 'Cov';
        title 'Estimated Covariance Matrix';
run;

/* merge survival estimates and stderrors with pred dataset */

data table;
        merge &pred survival sesurv ;
proc print data = table noobs;
        title 'Estimated Survival Probabilities';
run;
%mend;
```

18.2 The Macro CHECKDIST

```
%macro chekdist(data = _last_ , time = , cens = , censvals = 0 ,
                model = , pi = ) ;
%if "&model" = "exp" %then %do;
        proc lifetest data = &data noprint plots = (ls)  graphics;
                time &time*&cens(&censvals);
        %end;
%if "&model" = "weibull" %then %do;
        proc lifetest data = &data noprint plots = (lls) graphics;
                time &time*&cens(&censvals);
        %end;
%if "&model" ne "weibull" and "&model" ne "exp" %then %do;
        proc lifetest data = &data noprint outs = out;
                time &time*&cens(&censvals);
                axis1 label = (a = 90);
        %end;
%if "&model" = "lognorm" %then %do;
        data;
                set out;
                x = log(t);
                y = -probit(survival);
                label x = 'log(t)';
                label y = '-probit(survival)';
        proc gplot;
                plot y*x /vaxis = axis1;
        %end;
%if "&model" = "expcure" %then %do;
        data;
                set out;
                do pi = &pi ;
                y = log((survival - pi)/(1 - pi));
                output;
        end;
        label y = 'log[(survival-pi)/(1-pi)]';
        %end;
```

```
%if "&model" = "gomp" %then %do;
      data;
              set out;
              do pi = &pi;
              y=log(1-log(survival)/log(pi));
              output;
              end;
              label y = 'log[1-log(survival)/log(pi)]';
              %end;
%if "&model" = "gomp" or "&model" = "expcure" %then %do;
      proc gplot;
              plot y*t = pi /vaxis = axis1;
              %end;
%mend;
```

References

Altman, D. G., Lausen, B., Sauerbrei, W., Schumacher, M. (1994), "Dangers of Using 'optimal' Cutpoints in the Evaluation of Prognostic Factors," *Journal of the National Cancer Institute*, 86, 829-35.

Bowman, L. C., Castleberry, R. P., Cantor, A. B., Joshi, V. V., Cohn, S., Smith, E., Yu, A. L., Brodeur, G. M., Hayes, F., and Look, A., "Genetic Staging of Unresectable or Metastatic Neuroblastoma in Infants: a Pediatric Oncology Group Study," *Journal of the National Cancer Institute* (in press).

Breslow, N. (1970), "A Generalized Kruskal-Wallis Test for Comparing K Samples Subject to Unequal Patterns of Censorship," *Biometrika*, 57, 579-594.

Breslow, N. E. (1974), "Covariance Analysis of Censored Survival Data," *Biometrics*, 30, 89-99.

Cantor, A. B. (1992), "Sample Size Calculations for the Log Rank Test: A Gompertz Model Approach," *Journal of Clinical Epidemiology*, 45, 1131-1136.

Cantor, A. B. (1994), "A Test of the Association of a Time-Dependent State Variable to Survival," *Computer Methods and Programs in Biomedicine*, 46, 101-105.

Cantor, A. B. and Shuster, J. J. (1992), "Parametric Versus Non-Parametric Methods for Estimating Cure Rates Based on Censored Survival Data," *Statistics in Medicine*, 11, 931- 937.

Cantor, A. B. and Shuster, J. J. (1994), "Re: Dangers of Using 'optimal' Cutpoints in the Evaluation of Prognostic Factors [letter]," *Journal of the National Cancer Institute*, 86, 1798-1799.

Cox, D. R. (1972), "Regression Models and Life Tables," *Journal of the Royal Statistical Society*, B, 34, 187-220.

Crowley, J. (1974), "Asymptotic Normality of a New Non-Parametric Statistic for Use in Organ Transplant Studies," *Journal of the American Statistical Association*, 69, 1006-1011.

Gamel J. W., Vogel, R. L., Valagussa, P., and Bonadonna G. (1994), "Parametric Survival Analysis of Adjuvant Therapy for Stage II Breast Cancer," *Cancer*, 74, 2483-90.

Garg, M. L., Rao, B. R., Redmond, C. K. (1970), "Maximum Likelihood Estimation of the Parameters of the Gompertz Survival Function," *Applied Statistics*, 19, 152-159.

Gehan, E. A. (1965), "A Generalized Wilcoxon Test for Comparing Arbitrarily Singly-censored Samples," *Biometrika*, 52, 203-223.

Gehan, E. A. and Siddiqui, M. M. (1973), "Simple Regression Methods for Survival Time Studies," *Journal of the American Statistical Association*, 68, 848-856.

George, S. L. and Desu, M. M. (1974), "Planning the Size and Duration of a Clinical Trial: Studying the Time to Some Critical Event," *Journal of Chronic Diseases*, 27, 15-24.

Goldman, A.I. (1984), "Survivorship Analysis When Cure Is a Possibility: A Monte Carlo Study," *Statistics in Medicine*, 3, 153-163.

Gompertz, B. (1825), "On the Nature of the Function Expressive of the Law of Human Mortality, and on the New Mode of Determining the Value of Life Contingencies," *Philosophical Transactions of the Royal Society*, Series A, 115, 513-580.

Gray, R. J. and Tsiatis, A. A. (1989), "A Linear Rank Test for Use When the Main Interest Is in Cure Rates," *Biometrics*, 45, 899-904.

Greenwood, M. (1926), "The Natural Duration of Cancer," *Reports on Public Health and Medical Subjects*, 33, London: Her Majesty's Stationary Office, 1-26.

Hall, W. J., and Wellner, J. A. (1980), "Confidence Bands for a Survival Curve from Censored Data," *Biometrika*, 97, 133-143.

Harrington, D. P. and Fleming, T. R. (1982), "A Class of Rank Test Procedures for Censored Survival Data," *Biometrika*, 69, 553-566.

Haybittle J. (1959), "The Estimation of the Proportion of Patients Cured After Treatment for Cancer of the Breast," *British Journal of Radiology*, 32, 725-733.

Kalbfleisch, J. D., and Prentice, R. L. (1980), *The Statistical Analysis of Failure Time Data*, New York: John Wiley and Sons.

Kaplan, E.L. and Meier, P.L. (1958), "Nonparametric Estimation from Incomplete Observations," *Journal of the American Statistical Association*, 53, 457-481.

Lachin, J. (1981), "Introduction to Sample Size Determination and Power Analysis for Clinical Trials," *Controlled Clinical Trials*, 2, 93-113.

Lakatos, E. (1988), "Sample Sizes Based on the Log-Rank Statistic in Complex Clinical Trials," *Biometrics*, 44, 229-241.

Laska, E. M. and Meisner, M. J. (1992), "Nonparametric Estimation and Testing in a Cure Model," *Biometrics*, 48, 1223-1234.

Lee, E. T., Desu, M. M., and Gehan, E. A. (1975), "A Monte Carlo Study of the Power of Some Two-sample Tests," *Biometrika*, 62, 425-432.

Look, A.T., Hayes, F. A., Shuster, J. J., Douglass, E. C., Castleberry, R. P., Bowman, L. C., Smith, E. I., and Brodeur, G. M. (1991), "Clinical Relevance of Tumor Cell Ploidy and N-myc Gene Amplification in Childhood Neuroblastoma: a Pediatric Oncology Group Study," *Journal of Clinical Oncology*, 9, 581-591.

Lui, K. J. (1992), "Sample Size Determination Under an Exponential Model in the Presence of a Confounder and Type I Censoring," *Controlled Clinical Trials*, 13, 446-458.

Liu, P. Y. and Dahlberg, S. (1995), "Design and Analysis of Multarm Clinical Trails with Survival Endpoints," *Controlled Clinical Trials*, 16, 119-130.

Makuch, R. W. and Simon R. M. (1982), "Sample Size Requirements for Comparing Time- to- Failure among k Treatment Groups," *Journal of Chronic Diseases*, 35, 861-867.

Mantel, N. (1966), "Evaluation of Survival Data and Two New Rank Order Statistics Arising in its Consideration," *Cancer Chemotherapy Reports*, 50, 163-170.

Mantel, N. and Byar, D. (1974), "Evaluation of Response Time Data Involving Transient States: An Illustration Using Heart-Transplant Data," *Journal of the American Statistical Association*, 69, 81-86.

Mantel, N. and Haenszel, W. (1959), "Statistical Aspects of the Analysis of Data from Retrospective Studies of Disease," *Journal of the National Cancer Institute*, 22, 719-748.

Miller, R. G. (1981), *Survival Analysis*, New York: Wiley.

Miller, R. G. (1983), "What Price Kaplan-Meier," *Biometrics,* 39, 1077-1081.

Nelson, W. (1969) "Hazard Plotting for Incomplete Failure Data," *Journal of Quality Technology*, 1, 27-25.

Oakes, D. (1993), "A Note on the Kaplan-Meier Estimator," *The American Statistician*, 47, 39-40.

Peto, R. (1973), "Experimental Survival Curves for Interval-censored Data," *Applied Statistics*, 22, 86-93.

Peto, R. and Peto, J. (1972), "Asymptotically Efficient Rank Invariant Test Procedures (with Discussion)," *Journal of the Royal Statistical Society*, A, 135, 185-206.

Peto, R., Pike, M. C., Armitage, P., Breslow, N. E., Cox, D. R., Howard, S. V., Mantel, N., McPherson, K., Peto, J., and Smith, P. G. (1977), "Design and Analysis of Randomized Clinical Trials Requiring Prolonged Observation of Each Patient: II Analyses and Examples," *British Journal of Cancer*, 35, 1-39.

Prentice, R. L. (1978), "Linear Rank Tests with Right Censored Data," *Biometrika*, 65, 167-179.

Prentice, R. L. and Marek, P. (1979), "A Qualitative Discrepency Between Censored Data Rank Tests," *Biometrics*, 35, 861-867.

Reid, N. M. (1981), "Influence Functions for Censored Data," *Annals of Statistics,* 9, 78-92.

Riley, W. J., Maclaren, N. K., Krischer, J. P., Spillar, R. P., Silverstein, J. H., Schatz, D. A., Schwartz, S., Malone, J., Shah, S., Vadheim, C., and Rotter, J. I. (1990), "A Prospective Study of the Development of Diabetes in Relatives of Patients with Insulin Dependent Diabetes," *New England Journal of Medicine*," 323, 1167-1172.

Rubenstein, L. V., Gail, M. H., and Santner, T. J. (1981), "Planning the Duration of a Comparative Clinical Trial with Loss to Follow-up and a Period of Continued Observation," *Journal of Chronic Diseases*, 34, 469-479.

SAS Institute, Inc. (1996), *SAS/STAT Software: Changes and Enhancements through Release 6.11*, Cary NC, SAS Institute Inc., 813-814.

Sander, J. M. (1975), "Asymptotic Normality of Linear Combinations of Functions of Order Statistics with Censored Data," Technical Report #8, Division of Biostatistics, Stanford University, Stanford, California.

Shapiro, S., Venet, W., Strax, P., and Venet, L. (1988), *Periodic Screening for Breast Cancer: The Health Insurance Plan Project and Its Sequelae*, 1963-1986, Baltimore: The Johns Hopkins University Press.

Shih, J. H. (1995), "Sample Size Calculation for Complex Clinical Trials with Survival Endpoints," *Controlled Clinical Trials*, 16, 395-407.

Shuster, J. J. (1990), *Handbook of Sample Size Guidelines for Clinical Trials*, Boca Raton: CRC Press, Inc.

Sposto, R. and Sather, H.N. (1985), "Determining the Duration of Comparative Clinical Trials While Allowing for Cure," *Journal of Chronic Diseases*, 38, 683-690.

Tarone, R. and Ware, J. (1977), "On Distribution-free Tests for Equality of Survival Distributions," *Biometrika*, 64, 156-160.

Turnbull, B.W. (1976), "The Empirical Distribution Function from Arbitrarily Grouped, Censored and Truncated Data," *Journal of the Royal Statistical Society*, Series B, 38, 290-295.

Index

Call your local SAS® office to order these other books and tapes available through the Books by Users℠ program: